D0058927

Spice Up, Slim Down

A guide to adding spice to your diet to improve
health and lose weight

Melina B. Jampolis, MD

With Kristina Petersen, PhD

Cover Design by Jane Teis
Illustrations by Daniel Diaz

ISBN-10: 0692971319
ISBN-13: 978-0-692-97131-4
Library of Congress Control Number: 2017916978
Melina B. Jampolis MD A Prof Corp, Studio City, CA

DEDICATION

To my husband Benjamin, thank you for your unwavering support and enthusiasm for all of my endeavors and for trying to keep me (moderately) sane while helping to raise our two wonderful sons.

Spice Up, Slim Down

CONTENTS

Acknowledgments   i

Introduction   3

Ten Stars of the Spice World   9

Spice Blends, Trios, and Tips   45

Seven Ways to Slim Down with Spices   53

Spice Up, Slim Down Recipes   59

   Dressings, Dips, Sauces, Appetizers   59

   Entrees   63

   Soups and Sides   67

   Desserts and Baked Goods   72

Spice up, Slim Down Contributor Recipes   75

Conclusion   137

Personal Spice Notes   139

References   145

Recipe Index   159

Spice Up, Slim Down

ACKNOWLEDGMENTS

Writing a book is not easy and I had a lot of help making my vision for this book come to life. Thanks to Dr. Kristina Petersen for her extensive literature search into the health benefits of spices that helped shaped the first part of the book. Thanks to Chefs Sandra Mallut and Aaron Robbins for their delicious, spice-filled recipes. Thanks to Stacey Healey for her extensive help with the spice history research, simple spice uses, and administrative help and thanks to my assistant Andrea Tutone for helping out too wherever she could.

Thanks to writers Alice Kelly and Mary Mihaly for transforming my words into something that the reader could both enjoy and hopefully be inspired by. Special thanks to one of my dearest friends and a wonderful author herself Teresa Rodriguez for helping me pull everything together into a coherent and inviting format.

And finally, big thanks to all my friends, colleagues and experts who contributed recipes to this book – your support and enthusiasm for spices was very much appreciated and I'm extremely grateful to each and every one of you for your willingness to contribute.

Spice Up, Slim Down

INTRODUCTION

Let's face it: Some of the things we do to improve our health can be hard. Quitting smoking is hard. Losing lots of weight (and keeping it off) is hard. And getting up early to exercise when you'd rather snuggle under the covers can be hard, too. But I am thrilled to tell you that some healthy behaviors aren't hard at all. In fact, they're downright easy! One of the simplest of all is adding delicious, health-boosting spices to the foods you eat every day.

Spices add amazing taste and aroma to your meals. By providing bursts of complex flavor, they have the power to transform everyday foods from bland to exciting. Spices bring new tastes to foods, and when used correctly, they highlight the naturally delicious flavors that are already in the foods we eat.

It's not just about flavor, though. Spices can have a powerful impact on your health as well as your palate. Compounds found in spices have been associated with a range of important health benefits, including better heart and brain health, improved blood sugar control, lower levels of inflammation throughout your body, healthier bacteria in your gut, weight loss, and a lower risk of some kinds of cancer. Although the healing power of spices has been known for centuries, researchers are continuing to learn more about the ways in which spices can boost health.

Using spices truly is one of the easiest ways to improve your health. Adding a pinch of cinnamon to a cup of morning coffee, sprinkling fresh basil into a salad at lunch, or stirring turmeric and cumin into a zesty curry dinner are some of the easiest, most enjoyable ways I know of to help optimize your health and help you get—or stay—slim.

Food As Medicine

My interest in spices has grown out of my passion for using food as medicine. As a physician, I know that medicine has its place in treating and preventing disease. But as a board-certified physician nutrition specialist—one of only several hundred practicing in the United States—I understand that food can often be the best medicine of all. I specialize exclusively in using nutrition for weight loss and the prevention and treatment of disease, and any discussion of the healing power of foods must include spices, which are among the most potent health-supporting foods. In fact, in a recent analysis of over 1,100 foods, four of the top five foods highest in antioxidants—and 13 of the top 50--were spices.

By the way, when I talk about "spices" I am referring to what we usually think of as spices—the contents of the jars in your spice rack—as well as fresh and dried herbs. Generally, herbs come from the leaves of a plant, and spices come from the seed, root, stem, bark, fruit, or other part of a plant. For example, the herb cilantro comes from the leaves of the coriander plant, and the spice coriander comes from the plant's fruits, which look like seeds.

I was first exposed to the amazing potential of spices about eight years ago, when I was introduced to a weight-loss supplement containing capsaicin, an active compound found in chili peppers including cayenne. Weight loss is a health goal for many of my patients, so I was intrigued to learn about studies using capsaicin supplements to boost metabolism, burn fat, and increase feelings of fullness. I started having some success using capsaicin supplements

4

with my patients, but since I'm such a believer in food as medicine, my interest soon expanded beyond supplements and to the health benefits of the culinary spices we use in food.

Then, at a symposium sponsored by the National Institutes of Health a few years ago, I was completely blown away by a presentation about the potential health benefits of curcumin, the bioactive compound that gives the spice turmeric its bright yellow color. Researchers have discovered evidence that curcumin may have promising beneficial health effects on dozens of diseases, including cancer, cardiovascular disease, arthritis, Crohn's disease, ulcerative colitis, irritable bowel disease, dementia, diabetes, and many others. Even though I've built my professional career around the belief that food is our most powerful medicine, I was truly shocked to discover that this one spice could have so many health benefits. Then, as I learned about the potential power of other spices, I realized that I had to delve more into this topic.

How do spices boost health and help you slim down? There are a few mechanisms, which I'll explain in detail later in this book when I discuss individual spices, but in short, they contain powerful antioxidants that help protect your cells from damage, reduce inflammation, help with blood sugar control and insulin resistance (a condition in which your body does not respond appropriately to insulin which leads to excess insulin and weight gain – especially belly fat), and add flavor without calories. Using spices also helps reduce our reliance on salt, which is over consumed by 90 percent of Americans.

People who eat spices are, overall, healthier than those who don't. A fascinating 2015 study in China looked at the diets of nearly half a million people over four years. Compared with people who ate blander diets, the study found that people who ate spicier foods lived longer and had a lower incidence of cancer, heart disease, and respiratory diseases. The people who ate spicy foods almost every day had a 14 percent lower risk of dying during the four-year study than those who ate spicy foods less than once a week.

Spicing up your food is a great idea for so many reasons. Spices make food taste better, they can improve health, and they may even extend life. What's not to love about that?

Late To The Party

The funny thing is, we in the United States are some of the last ones in the world to understand and appreciate the incredible contributions spices can make to our health. Nearly every culture and country in the world has a rich history of using spices for health and flavor—except for the U.S., where the most used spices are salt (which is actually a mineral) and pepper. We don't realize how important spices are, and how revered they've been throughout the world for centuries. At certain times in history, spices were considered more valuable than gold, and countries went to war over them.

I've also discovered that most Americans are pretty much clueless when it comes to using spices. And that included me, until recently. We sprinkle cinnamon on our oatmeal, enjoy basil on gourmet pizza, and line up for pumpkin-spice lattes in the Fall. But overall, we don't know which spices to use, how to use them, or which foods to use them with.

That's why I wrote this book. I want all of us—myself included—to learn how to use spices regularly to optimize their impact. This book is for my patients and all the people who want to spice up their health without spending hours in the kitchen laboring over complicated recipes with lengthy ingredient lists.

Before we go any further, though, I want to put my cards on the table. The truth is, I'm pretty clueless in the kitchen. My mother is an amazing cook, and I spent part of my childhood in France, surrounded by astonishingly delicious food. Despite my upbringing, though, I am a terrible cook. When I first became interested in spicing up my food, I was completely intimidated. Reading complicated recipes with long lists of ingredients made me want to reach for a glass of wine and order takeout! I knew the only way for me to incorporate spices into my everyday meals would be if I could do it simply. That's why the focus of this book is to give you easy ways to spice up your diet. This book is as much for me as it is for you.

Spices, Simply

In the following pages, I'll tell you about 10 of the most powerful and commonly used spices, those that have the most potential for promoting good health and preventing disease, along with several honorable mentions that are less common or don't have quite as much research to support their health benefits but are still super healthful and delicious. And I'll share some of the exciting ways that spices help with weight loss, heart health, brain health, diabetes management, gut health, and other disease prevention.

I'll also provide an array of relatively simple recipes that use the spices I feature in this book, as well as tips for incorporating spices into your everyday meals. I've hit up dozens of my favorite celebrity chefs, nutritionists, personal trainers, authors, friends, and even an ultra-marathon runner, who have generously offered to share their favorite spice recipes. And again somewhat selfishly, I've even include advice for wine-pairing ideas for foods that contain spices.

If you don't have a clue how to use spices in food—other than sprinkling salt and pepper on your steak and cinnamon on your toast—don't worry. I'm going to give you dozens of ideas about how to use health-promoting spices. You can do this, even if you're as clueless as I am in the kitchen.

I'll also show you how easy it is to use spices and herbs in your kitchen. Good ground spices aren't necessarily cheap, but if stored correctly they last a long time and a little goes a long way in many cases. And fresh herbs are easier than ever to keep on hand—I buy fresh basil plants at Trader Joe's, set them on my kitchen windowsill, and snip off leaves whenever I need them. (OK, full confession—my husband does the snipping, but I did buy the basil plant!) Talk about accessible.

Don't worry if you're not a big from-scratch cook. You can add spices to quick-prep foods, such as smoothies, salads, sandwiches, and frozen meals you heat up in the microwave. You can even sprinkle them on prepared foods you pick up from restaurants or grocery stores. Think of this book as a user's manual for integrating spices into your diet no matter what kind of a cook you are (or aren't).

And, although this isn't a diet book, it does contain advice for readers who want to improve the quality of their diet or take off excess weight. I'll tell you all about how spices can play an important role in weight loss and healthy weight maintenance.

Once you read the simple guidelines in this book, you'll be ready to start spicing up your life, adding wonderful flavors to your food, and taking full advantage of the many health benefits that spices can bring to your table.

TEN STARS OF THE SPICE WORLD

I may not be an experienced chef, but I know about flavor. These 10 spice stars were easy to choose because all of them are in my cupboard right now, and I'll bet they're in yours, too. There's a reason for that: we reach for these spices, more than almost any others you can name. I've included them here because they boost our health and we use most of them almost daily – though some are super- healthy and I think they should be even more popular! Some of these spices add zest, depth and great flavor to our food – but even if they're a little challenging flavor-wise, they add so much to our well-being that finding a way to add them to our meals is totally worth it!

I love spice-rich foods, but they don't just taste good; they're also packed with antioxidants and other components that help keep us healthy. I've started the write-up for each spice with some fun history about it – we think of them as seasonings, but some were used as an aphrodisiac, a fabric dye, and even as a cure for gout!

Then, I give you the most updated science for each spice. This information shows you that the health benefits of spices are proven and real, so I hope the research will motivate you to incorporate more spices into your diet. Once you start eating spicier meals, you're bound to feel better, you may lose weight, and you will definitely get closer to your other health goals. In the next section, I'll give more details and specifics about using spices to lose weight.

KEY TO ILLUSTRATIONS OF SPICE BENEFITS

ARTHRITIS

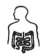

GUT HEALTH

INSULIN RESISTANCE

HIGH CHOLESTEROL

BRAIN HEALTH

HIGH BLOOD PRESSURE

CANCER

INFLAMMATION

DIABETES

METABOLISM

These spices are the top performers, ready for prime time!

Cinnamon – The diabetes destroyer

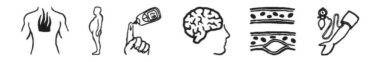

Does anyone not remember eating cinnamon toast as a kid? I'm not talking about toast made with that prefab "cinnamon bread" or "cinnamon swirl" from the supermarket. I mean the real deal – white bread toasted, buttered with real butter, and covered with sugar and cinnamon powder sprinkled from a can. The kind of cinnamon toast that instantly puts you in your mom's kitchen again, without a care in the world. My mom used to make us cinnamon toast on Saturday mornings in winter, before we went skiing. As food memories go, it's heavenly – if not particularly healthy!

Cinnamon is the most popular spice, yet few people know there are two varieties: Cassia, which we get from China, and Ceylon cinnamon from Sri Lanka (formerly called Ceylon).

Both types have been around for centuries, though we didn't always flavor our food with them. The Egyptians used fragrant cinnamon as a perfuming agent in the embalming process, and the Old Testament mentions it as an ingredient in oil used for religious ceremonies. Chinese healers in ancient times made it a part of Traditional Chinese Medicine for treating muscle aches and respiratory conditions, and Ayurvedic practitioners in India used it to remedy muscle spasms, respiratory problems (flu, coughs, chest congestion), stomach issues and diabetes. Along the way, healers also discovered it helps fight infections.

Because it had to be transported over rugged terrain for thousands of miles, in Europe it was rare and so expensive that in order to justify their exorbitant prices, traders concocted bizarre myths about the spice's origins. Still, it was highly desired – partly because it was an effective way to preserve meat in those pre-refrigeration days – so aristocrats bought it.

Today, of course, it's cinnamon's taste that has us hooked. We see it everywhere – in recipes for baked goods, on our oatmeal, in smoothies and baked fruits, even in martinis! But now also there's plenty of fresh evidence that it's good for our health. For starters, a review of 10 studies published in *Annals of Family Medicine* showed that cinnamon lowers fasting glucose levels – meaning, the sugar/glucose level in your system before you eat anything – in diabetic patients. Other studies showed the same effect on healthy people who eat cinnamon with a meal, which makes the spice a great weapon against getting diabetes in the first place.

And scientists recently learned that whether you're at your goal weight or need to lose some pounds, simply sprinkling cinnamon on your cereal each morning will lower your blood sugar concentration. That same study showed that people in a range of body weights also see more insulin sensitivity, so the insulin your body creates naturally can do its job more effectively.

Research also shows that eating up to 6 grams of cinnamon each day (a little over a teaspoon) lowers LDL cholesterol (the "bad" cholesterol) and triglycerides ("blood fat"). As an added bonus, it raises HDL ("good") cholesterol in people with diabetes.

Another advantage to eating cinnamon is that it lowers blood pressure in people diagnosed with prediabetes and type 2 diabetes. A clinical trial showed that just by eating less than half a teaspoon per day, those patients were able to lower both their systolic and diastolic blood pressure (basically defined as pressure on the ventricles of the heart as blood pumps through it).

And here's a cinnamon benefit that people with all sorts of conditions can appreciate: this dynamite spice also combats inflammation, a condition we learn more about all the time. What we know is, even though acute, short term inflammation helps enable us to battle injury and infections, long term (also known as chronic) inflammation can damage our joints and hurt our heart, lungs, skin and even affect our mental health. So when it comes to chronic inflammation, less is more!

Cinnamon also contains powerful antioxidants – our best weapon against cancer- and illness-causing molecules called free radicals – so the logical conclusion is that cinnamon may help to fight many illnesses brought on by free radicals, including cancer.

Lastly, cinnamon just might make us smarter! When scientists publishing in the journal *Nutrition Research* studied people aged 60 and older who had prediabetes, they found that cinnamon eaters had better memory function. Other research shows that it could prevent Alzheimer's and dementia from developing, or stop those disorders in their early stages. Animals in the lab have demonstrated that cinnamon may slow brain-changes that trigger Alzheimer's disease and correct the mental decline caused by the disease. That benefit alone is enough to keep me sprinkling it on everything!

When you go to purchase cinnamon, look for the Ceylon variety. Its bark is darker and richer-looking – with a higher price tag to match – but experts claim it has more healing power. How do you get cinnamon into your diet? It really couldn't be easier – as I mentioned earlier, just sprinkle a little on your oatmeal or yogurt. You also can add it to chili, baked goods, sauces and smoothies. One of my favorite ways of incorporating cinnamon into my diet is simply stirring it into my morning coffee – I love that taste! I also always put in in my yogurt (usually with a little stevia and a tablespoon or two of nuts or seeds). And when I bake breakfast muffins or pancakes for my kids (when I have time), I always throw some into the mix.

Turmeric – The anti-inflammatory rock star

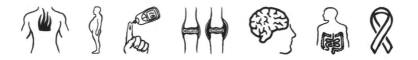

This one just might be the all-star of spices! Turmeric is another ancient spice-dynamo used to treat more than 60 diseases across the centuries. For more than 4,500 years, healers in Ayurvedic, Traditional Chinese Medicine and folk medicine put turmeric to work fighting congestion, inflammatory conditions, indigestion, chicken pox, shingles, measles, skin ailments, stress, colds and dozens more afflictions. And its amber hue makes it one of the prettiest spices – in fact, it used to be called the "poor man's saffron," named after the pricey (but healthy) Mediterranean spice, because of its golden-orange color!

Curcumin (not to be confused with cumin, another spice altogether that we'll tackle later in this section), is the active ingredient in turmeric, and it's the component of turmeric that delivers the most healing power. You might see the words "turmeric" and "curcumin" used interchangeably but they aren't exactly the same – turmeric is the spice that I want you to start including in your diet today. But if you're really trying to zero in on a specific health issue or have a specific health concern, you may also want to take a supplement containing curcumin, the more concentrated, potent ingredient.

Most of the research presented involves supplements containing curcumin because the more concentrated form produces more measurable results, but both are important for optimal health.

The turmeric plant is about three feet tall; like ginger, the part we use is the rhizome, or root. It even looks somewhat like ginger, gnarly and bumpy. India is the largest producer, but it's a kitchen staple across Asia; in Northern Africa you'll find it in stews and tagines –

dishes named after the funnel-shaped clay pot they're cooked in.

As a health booster, turmeric can claim the major "anti's," antioxidant and anti-inflammatory – more than almost any other spice – so it's a mighty weapon against some of our most serious diseases. Inflammation plays a critical role in heart disease, and cell research has shown that turmeric both lowers inflammatory molecules and increases anti-inflammatory molecules. Reducing inflammation is a great benefit; it helps protect blood vessels in the heart and the brain from damage.

Animal studies also found that taking turmeric supplements is associated with less plaque (fat buildup) in blood vessels, and similar findings of healthier blood vessels have been found in studies of humans taking turmeric – thus further lowering their risk of heart disease. Another study found that postmenopausal women who supplemented their diets with curcumin each day for just eight weeks likewise had healthier blood vessels. And in one study in which the human subjects took curcumin daily for six months, participants not only reduced the stiffness in their arteries, they also lost about 5 percent of body fat and an inch off of their waists!

Curcumin is effective against arthritis pain and gastrointestinal disorders, too. Both conditions relate to inflammation, and an analysis of eight studies showed people who took curcumin felt less pain from arthritis after 8 to 12 weeks. Other studies of cells and animals found curcumin reduced gut inflammation, and it also worked with the intestinal wall to help prevent leaky gut. And for people whose guts are healthy, studies have found that turmeric's anti-microbial power slows the growth of harmful bacteria in the gut.

Research suggests that turmeric also affects our brain health in a significant way. Here in the U.S. we see four times as many cases of Alzheimer's disease as in India, and some experts believe it's because curry is such a major part of Indian cuisine – and turmeric (along with cumin, another "top 10" spice) is a primary ingredient in curry powder. In a study conducted in Singapore, people who regularly ate curry showed better brain function than those who never ate curry, or ate it rarely. Those conclusions are supported by cell and animal studies that prove curcumin reduces the levels of inflammatory molecules that may contribute to Alzheimer's disease and dementia. Curcumin also improves blood flow to the brain and increases levels of a protein that supports the maintenance and growth of brain cells and the pathways that connect them.

Can you see why I say turmeric is the most important spice to eat regularly?

Very few studies have directly investigated the effect of curcumin on cognitive function, so we need more research in this area. But one study showed that people aged 60 to 85 years who took curcumin daily for four weeks did improve their memories and mood. There's also evidence to suggest that curcumin might help ease symptoms of depression: according to an analysis of six studies, people diagnosed with depression who took curcumin every day reduced their depressive symptoms.

Luckily, it's not too challenging to get turmeric into your diet. Since turmeric is a main ingredient in curry, you get turmeric's abundance of health benefits every time you eat a curry dish (just limit the heavy cream and super oily curry dishes). Simply add curry powder – sold at any supermarket – to soups, stews, chili, omelets, sauces, marinades and curried vegetable dishes, or to meat, chicken or fish rubs.

You can dress up a bowl of plain-looking brown rice – and add a slew of health benefits – by stirring in a little dried turmeric. Or try mixing in ¼ to ½ teaspoon when you bake, or even in your morning smoothie, to add that vibrant color to sweet dishes and make them healthier. But start with just a little bit and experiment; turmeric has its own flavor and it can change the way your food tastes.

Cayenne Pepper (aka chili pepper, red pepper)
The metabolism whisperer

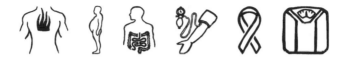

Here's another spice that's been around for thousands of years – 7,000, roughly. Historians think chili peppers originated in Bolivia and part of Brazil, then birds ate the seeds and deposited them throughout the Americas. They got to be a "hot item" because of something called capsaicin – the substance that puts the "hot" in "hot peppers" and the active ingredient in the spice we know as cayenne pepper.

Before the rest of the world discovered peppers, the Aztecs used them for cooking and religious rituals. But we can partly thank Christopher Columbus and his physician, Diego Alvarez Chanca, for hot peppers' worldwide popularity after they carried them home to Europe.

It seemed that each time people in a different country used cayenne peppers as medicine, they discovered a new health benefit from the peppers' capsaicin. Native Americans used to rub the peppers on their gums when they had a toothache. Overseas in Russia, Greece and Italy, people steeped peppers in vodka and drank it as a tonic. In the West Indies, some healers still give cayenne to fight yellow fever.

Although like most spices cayenne was used for treating a range of ailments over the centuries, its most exciting modern day feature by far is its ability to speed up your metabolism, increase fat burning and shrink your appetite. (Translation: it can help you slim down!)

And the research is pretty convincing: in two large reviews (a review is when researchers combine several studies looking at the same factor, in this case capsaicin intake), they found that participants in 13 of the studies burned more calories when they ate foods containing capsaicin – sometimes after eating a hot pepper, or even a sweet pepper, in just one meal. But sweet peppers only contain a small amount of capsaicin, so if you really want to speed up your metabolism, reach for the hotter varieties.

In the same two reviews, seven out of 11 studies found that people who were given capsaicin burned more fat and lowered body fat stores. (In case you were wondering, the other four studies only looked at metabolism.) And five of those seven studies showed that capsaicin reduces appetite, so those in the group consuming capsaicin ate smaller portions than the non-capsaicin-consumers, even though they were told to go ahead and eat whatever they liked.

Another way cayenne pepper might help long-term weight control is its effect on "good" gut bacteria. A cell study found that it stimulated their growth – and when the same healthy bacterial growth was found in a study of animals who were fed high-fat food and capsaicin, the animals lost weight in spite of their diets. A bonus of that study: their blood sugar levels improved, too.

Can hot peppers help you live longer?

One of the most fascinating potential health benefits of capsaicin is that it might actually help us live longer. Cayenne is one of the main foods that the Hunza people in northern Pakistan eat, and they typically live for more than a century. Researchers also have seen that it lowers our risk of dying from a number of deadly diseases, including cancer and diseases of the heart and lungs. And as I mentioned earlier, in China, a huge study found that people who ate spicy foods most days had a 14 percent lower risk of dying from any cause than individuals who ate it less than once a week. That conclusion held true regardless of the type of spicy foods they ate – fresh or dried chili peppers, chili sauce or chili oil.

And capsaicin couldn't be easier to add to your diet. Just sprinkle a little cayenne pepper in soups, chilies, home-made spice rubs, and even desserts. If you aren't used to eating spicy food, start slowly as cayenne pepper is very potent and can burn your mouth (like any raw hot pepper or hot sauce).

I have grown to love spicy foods as I get older – which is a good thing since metabolism drops with age. I add cayenne to a lot of foods – I even drink it in lemon water with a little stevia when I'm really trying to slim down. But if you buy ground cayenne at the store and add it to a drink, be sure to keep stirring because it doesn't dissolve well.

I also love to combine cayenne with other spices – in fact my favorite recipe (Spiced Butternut Squash) from my last book, combines cayenne pepper with cumin, coriander, cinnamon, onion powder. I included lots of amazing cayenne recipes in this book too, so you have lots of options for reaping the benefits .

Red pepper flakes (the kind you might put on pizza) also contain capsaicin so feel free to add them to your cooking, too. (Just don't load up on pizza, as any metabolic benefit will be offset by the calories in the pizza!) You can also find a little cayenne in chili powder, which I talk about in the section on blends. Because chili powder contains a smaller amount of cayenne, you may not get quite as many metabolic benefits, but it's even easier to use and contains lots of other healthful spices, so I alternate between both.

Ginger – The arthritis buster

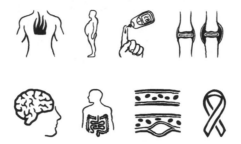

In the supermarket, you'll often come across fresh ginger, a knobby-looking root, among the vegetables in the produce section. It's another spice whose use has spanned thousands of years, and it's packed with so many powerful healing ingredients that it appears on most lists of "superfoods."

Ginger originated in southern China, later spreading to India (the largest producer today), the Middle East, the Roman Empire and the southern Caribbean. One of its most widespread uses was for treating nausea – that's why we reach for ginger ale when we have a "sour stomach!" In Myanmar (formerly Burma), practitioners mix it with local plants as a flu preventative, and in the Congo they add it to sap from the mango tree – a simple concoction they believe is a cure-all.

We have easy access to the spice now, but historically ginger was considered a luxury. In the 13th and 14th centuries, a pound of ginger root could be traded for a sheep. Eventually, preserved ginger made its way into dessert recipes for the rich and famous, and royalty joined in: Queen Elizabeth I is recognized as the creator of the "gingerbread man."

Today we consume ginger fresh, powdered, dried, in juices, as a tea, candied and in curries and oil. And we don't just eat and drink it; because it soothes and helps heal us, ginger also appears on the ingredients lists of perfumes, cosmetics and skin creams. With so many options, spicing up your life with ginger is easy.

And it's well worth keeping in your kitchen, especially if you have arthritis. It turns out ginger's most powerful health bonus is its ability to reduce inflammation – and if you have joint pain, inflammation is the culprit. In an analysis of five studies, researchers checked participants' CRP (C-reactive protein, a measure of inflammation in the body) and the group taking ginger reduced their "whole body inflammation" significantly. A review of five more studies found that ginger went a long way in relieving pain and disability in people who'd been diagnosed with osteoarthritis.

The list of ginger's health benefits goes on, and one of the most important is its ability to decrease insulin resistance, a dangerous condition in which the body doesn't utilize insulin correctly. Four studies of people with type 2 diabetes have confirmed ginger as a potent insulin-resistance warrior.

We also know ginger can lower cholesterol and blood glucose (sugar) levels. No less than nine studies proved that people who took ginger supplements for two to three months reduced their LDL ("bad") cholesterol and triglycerides, or "blood fat". They also raised their HDL, or "good" cholesterol levels.

Experiments also have shown that ginger is a "prebiotic," or substance that helps us grow friendly microorganisms in our intestines. It's an antibiotic, too – another factor that makes it useful against infections that can cause nausea.

And if you don't feel as mentally "sharp" as you'd like, there's some evidence that ginger might improve cognitive function – your ability to reason, remember and think clearly. A study of middle-aged women who took ginger supplements for two months reported that their attention spans and memories had improved.

Dried ginger is the easiest kind to use, and getting it into your diet couldn't be easier: it tastes great in smoothies (especially along with fresh or frozen peaches). Or, you can use it to add some zing to your oatmeal, yogurt and baked goods – just like cinnamon.

You can even make a tasty, soothing tea with dried ginger; just add ¼ teaspoon to a cup of boiling water. And if you have a sore joint, soak a washcloth in that tea and lay it on the painful spot, then cover it with a towel and hot water bottle for 20 minutes. You'll notice the difference.

Rosemary – The cancer protector

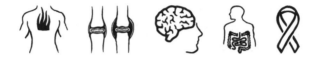

This spice's history is all about drama – a little surprising, since it's such a comforting sort of spice, maybe because we often serve it with comfort food, like beef roasts.

But eons ago, rosemary was all about love and death. It represented fidelity to the Greeks and Romans, and sprigs of rosemary were placed in bridal bouquets. The newlyweds took a few sprigs to their marital home and, before the sun went down on their wedding day, they planted some rosemary together. An old ballad captured the tradition: "Young men and maids do ready stand/With sweet rosemary in their hands."

It followed people to their final ceremonies, too. According to legend, rosemary was tossed onto graves as the deceased were laid to rest, giving it the nickname, "herb of remembrance." You can find a long list of ways in which healers used rosemary over the years. One of the more interesting was devised by Queen Isabella of Hungary, who concocted an alcohol extract from rosemary to treat her gout.

Others burned the spice in sick chambers, churches and courtrooms to purify the air and kill germs. Later, people believed it improved their memories and, before refrigeration, it was used to preserve meats.

It even had cosmetic value: people rubbed rosemary water into their skin, believing it could return their vigor and youth. Even Napoleon was a fan; Josephine introduced him to baths and colognes, and he doused himself with rosemary-scented cologne after his bath each morning.

As with most spices, rosemary is antioxidant powerhouse. It fights inflammation, too: in one clinical trial, people reduced their harmful inflammation levels after taking rosemary powder for just seven days, thanks to one of its most active ingredients, rosmarinic acid. Both human and animal studies have shown that this anti-inflammatory effect may help decrease the pain associated with arthritis. It also acts as a probiotic, like several other spices that contain rosmarinic acid, and may even help with ulcer healing according to one study.

Rosemary also helps us develop healthy blood vessels, and we don't have to be elderly or sick to enjoy this benefit. When researchers gave rosemary supplements to young, healthy individuals for 21 days, the number of participants with vascular conditions declined. The scientists suggested their improvements were likely due to rosemary's powerful antioxidants.

Rosemary even lowers blood sugar levels. In one study, animals that were fed rosemary supplements for three months cut their blood sugar levels by 12 percent. Those that had diabetes reduced their blood sugar by a whopping 45 percent, after only one month of supplements. We haven't yet investigated rosemary's effect on human glucose levels, but we do know from cell studies that rosemary activates molecules that help control glucose.

One of the most exciting properties of rosemary is its potential to neutralize cancer causing chemicals. One study in particular produced remarkable results: researchers added some rosemary to meat before grilling it at high temperatures – an activity that creates cancer-causing chemicals. But adding the rosemary before grilling the meat lowered the amount of those deadly chemicals by more than 70 percent! Both lab and animal studies also show that rosemary might also protect the skin from ultraviolet radiation which could decrease the risk of skin cancer and premature skin aging (age spots, wrinkles, and sagging skin).

And aside from its impact on brain diseases, rosemary might also boost normal brain functioning. In a study of healthy adults averaging 75 years in age, the group who were fed rosemary recalled information more quickly than those who didn't eat the herb – and that effect lasted up to six hours after they ate it. We've also seen rosemary improve thinking ability; in one study of animals that had suffered mild brain injuries, giving them rosemary extract raised their cognitive powers. In another animal study, the group that was fed rosemary extract for 28 days improved their long-term memories – all supporting the theory that rosemary does, indeed, help fight neurogenerative diseases.

Not surprisingly, rosemary is my favorite spice to add when I'm grilling any protein – meats, chicken, fish – and vegetables. Sometimes I toss in sprigs or needles; other times I blend the spice into a rub or marinade.

Rosemary also is an ingredient in Herbs de Provence, one of the spice blends I discuss later, but you can add it to almost any sauce, soup, marinade or olive oil-based dressing as well. The absolute simplest use (and one of the tastiest in my opinion) is to sprinkle rosemary on chicken with a little olive oil and grill it – easy peasy!

Oregano – The gut hero

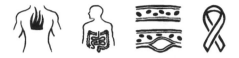

Say "oregano" and right away I think of homemade meatballs and tomato sauce, simmering on the stove, waiting to top a mountain of spaghetti.

But oregano isn't Italian at all. It's originally from Greece, and the ancient Greeks got creative about using it as a medicine. Hippocrates used it to treat stomach and breathing disorders; others in that era thought it was a remedy for poison (though it's not clear what would have been poisoning people back then). They also used it for treating edema (what you have when your feet swell up, once called "dropsy"), skin infections and even convulsions. And according to legend, the Greek goddess Aphrodite considered oregano a symbol of joy and grew it in her garden on Mount Olympus.

By the Middle Ages, people were chewing oregano to cure everything from rheumatism, toothaches, and indigestion to coughing fits. In China it was used for stomach disorders and fever. Today, oregano is a popular Turkish spice; more oregano is grown there than in any other country. Turkish cooks steep it to make oregano tea and water.

As part of my spice "prescription" for optimal health, oregano is the powerhouse spice for the gut; it helps promote the growth of the good bacteria that improves our health, and keeps the unhealthy bacteria from flourishing. Oregano is also a potent weapon against many of the bacteria that cause food poisoning and it may also help eradicate the H. pylori, the bacteria responsible for ulcers in many people. It may also help fight colon cancer – a test tube study found that an oregano extract, at levels found in the Mediterranean diet, killed cancer cells.

Oregano is also a forceful antioxidant; in a 2006 study it ranked second in antioxidant concentration (by weight) out of 1113 U.S. food samples. And it can help fight inflammation: in another study, it slowed the production of inflammatory molecules by a whopping 25 percent! That means it could lower the risk of diseases triggered by oxidative damage and inflammation, including heart disease and cancer.

There are a slew of other proven health benefits, too. In one study, people who were given oregano for three months raised their HDL cholesterol (the good kind), reduced the LDL/bad cholesterol, and had healthier blood vessels. Other studies show oregano reduces blood sugar and blood pressure, and even lowers cholesterol levels.

This flavorful spice is often found in Italian seasoning blends and pairs well with meat dishes, tomato-based dishes and eggs. Try adding it to store-bought sauces, soups and spreads to boost the health value of ready-made meals (even if the product already claims to have oregano, an extra boost can't hurt!). It might be especially important to eat oregano if you have digestive issues or if you have taken antibiotics recently.

Oregano is a wonderful addition to tomato-based soups and sauces. It also adds a touch of extra flavor to chicken, fish and even beans – just sprinkle a little on top! And oregano is a great addition to meatballs or burgers (just stick with lean cuts of red meat for optimal health).

Cumin – The belly buster

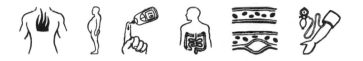

First, let's get clear so we're not confused: cumin and curcumin are not the same thing! Cumin is a spice and curcumin is the active ingredient in turmeric. Both are key ingredients in curry, that wonderful spice blend that's so important in Asian and Indian cooking.

Throughout history, cumin was always valuable, if not a downright luxury. Egyptians used it in mummifying their pharaohs, and the Bible refers to worshippers giving it to priests as their tithes. The Greeks even counted it as currency, and they used it to pay their taxes.

But cumin also has its romantic side. Long ago, wedding guests carried cumin in their pockets as a symbol of love and fidelity; some societies sent their soldiers to war with cumin bread. Arabs believed that ground cumin, honey and pepper could work as an aphrodisiac.

What has endured, though, is its beneficial impact on cardiometabolic diseases (like heart disease and diabetes)– it improves cholesterol levels, helps control blood sugar, helps you lose weight (especially belly fat) and, importantly, it decreases insulin resistance. All of those benefits are good news for people with pre-diabetes, diabetes, or metabolic syndrome (a common syndrome in those struggling with excess weight that includes at least three of the following: high blood sugar, high blood pressure, high triglycerides, low HDL (that is, not enough of the good cholesterol), and increased waist size). Cumin may even lower the risk of certain types of cancer.

And that impact on slimming down is significant. In one study of overweight adults, everyone received weight loss counseling but only one group also ate cumin. The results were impressive: after three months, the cumin-eaters lost almost 8 percent of their body weight, while the non-cumin group lost only 5.5 percent.

Cumin has shown other health benefits over the years. In folk medicine, people ground the seeds to make a drink that would help relieve flatulence, indigestion and other intestinal disorders. More recently, a number of animal studies show that cumin increases the secretion of digestive enzymes and molecules needed for digestion. This reduces food transit time (the overall digestive process), which has been associated with a lower risk of developing colon cancer.

A little cumin trivia

You already know that cumin figures into the cuisines of Mexico, India and North Africa (think Morocco and Egypt) in a major way; people in those lands use it daily to add color and flavor to their dishes. What you may not know is, cumin is the most popular spice in Mexican cooking and, just behind black pepper, it's the second-most popular spice in the world.

I happen to love cumin because it's so handy when I'm too lazy to cook from scratch (which is more often than I care to admit!). One of my favorite tricks is tossing some store-bought cumin into pre-made chili, along with an extra can of diced tomatoes, for an amazing upgrade in the flavor (and reduction in calories with the extra vegetables). And if I'm only snacking or need an easy appetizer, I'm currently obsessed with adding a pinch or two of cumin to my guacamole; that way I get terrific flavor plus the outstanding effect on my blood sugar and cholesterol levels.

Thyme – The brain and gut booster

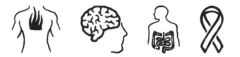

Thyme is a fascinating spice, partly because fables and mysticism, mixed with functionality, guided its history. People started using it some 5,000 years ago when the Ancient Egyptians discovered it relieved pain – but they also used it in embalming, believing it would smooth their passage into the afterlife.

The Romans, too, mixed their practical application (an antidote for poison) with symbolism; to them thyme signified respect, bravery, strength and courage. That belief carried into the Middle Ages, when thyme was a popular gift for men marching into battle. In the 1340s, realism took over as hordes of people, fearful of the Black Plague, used it to protect themselves from the epidemic and for treating plague-blistered skin.

By the 19th century, in the frilly Victorian era, the fairy-tale image of thyme came back to match the romantic notions of the day: people believed that a patch of wild thyme in the woods was created by fairies dancing on that spot. Little girls would camp out nearby, hoping to catch a glimpse of the fairies.

But science had evolved enough that we also began to see its role in medicine, particularly as a champion antioxidant and antibiotic. Already healers were covering wounds with bandages soaked in thyme and water to ward off infection. They also used it to remedy consumption, whooping cough and even nightmares and shyness.

Modern research supports many of those early beliefs. Like many other spices, thyme is both a potent antioxidant and a tenacious inflammation-fighter – it slows the production of inflammatory molecules while it speeds up production of those that fight inflammation. Animal studies have found that by doing both, it may reduce damage to our cells and organs and could help keep cancer cells and tumors from developing.

That same anti-inflammatory quality benefits our guts, too. Research shows that by reducing inflammation, thyme helps protect the gut wall and may help prevent leaky gut syndrome, a somewhat controversial diagnosis in mainstream medicine that may cause symptoms including bloating, gas, cramping, food sensitivities and joint pain. Another study found that it can help decrease the severity of colitis (inflammation of the bowel) and may help kill the H. pylori bacteria that is responsible for a majority of ulcers.

Like several other spices, thyme might help support brain health and reduce symptoms associated with Alzheimer's disease. In one study, mice were given a substance called thymol, which is one of the active ingredients in thyme, and 30 minutes later they were able to learn and think better than those who weren't given thymol. Thirty minutes! Research continues, but we definitely have reason to be optimistic about effective treatment and more importantly, prevention, of dementia. Spices, including thyme, could likely play an important role.

I love the way thyme tastes, so I use it a lot – and who doesn't need a little extra brain boost? For breakfast, it doesn't get easier than tossing a little thyme in with scrambled eggs and some goat cheese. (Thyme, by the way, is one of the best spices to pair with cheese. Ditto for dill and chives; they're all great with cheese.) And for dinner, I frequently roast cauliflower with thyme and olive oil – an amazing taste for about two minutes of prep work. By the way, I just learned that thyme comes in both powder form and dried leaf version – I prefer the dried leaf in my cooking but both are wonderful, healthy additions to your diet.

Coriander/Cilantro – The blood sugar busters

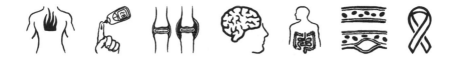

We think of them as two different spices, and from a culinary standpoint, they definitely are. But both come from the coriander plant: coriander is the seed, and cilantro, also known as "Chinese parsley," is the leaf.

We've been using it forever. Coriander was found in Tutankhamun's tomb; it was part of the pharaoh's royal sendoff because his subjects believed it was important food for the afterlife. That wasn't the only way the ancient Egyptians used coriander; they also thought it was an aphrodisiac. Two continents away, Asians were using it to treat stomach problems, and Ayurvedic physicians prescribed it as a diuretic. Over time, in other cultures, it was used as a folk remedy for vertigo, insomnia, high blood pressure, urinary tract infections, allergies and diabetes.

It's that last use – a treatment for diabetes – that endures as the mega-health benefit from eating coriander and cilantro. We know today that they help people with type 2 diabetes control their blood sugar, and they might lower blood sugar levels in healthy people as well. One study showed they can even help make blood vessels healthier and they're loaded with plenty of other health benefits, too – they help lower cholesterol and inflammation. In one animal study, coriander increased levels of healthy cholesterol and decreased levels of less healthy cholesterol.

In Germany, coriander is considered a safe and effective remedy for many digestive complaints. One study found that it was three times more effective than a placebo at relieving the abdominal pain in patients with irritable bowel syndrome (IBS). Another study found that it may help with constipation, and an animal study found that it helped relax digestive muscles, easing the discomfort of IBS.

Preliminary studies show that coriander and cilantro can have a healthy effect on the brain as well. In one animal study, both young and aged mice showed improved memory after being fed a diet that contained cilantro, and some animal studies have shown that coriander improves symptoms of Alzheimer's disease. Other mouse research showed that those effects might be passed on through breastfeeding; the offspring learned better after the mothers were given coriander seed extract

Cilantro is a great herb to use fresh since it adds so much flavor. It's especially tasty in Mexican and Asian dishes. You can add it to stir fry (towards the end, so the flavor stays), use it to top chili and soup, toss a little into rice dishes and dips for extra flavor and nutrition, and even chop it finely and blend it into salad dressing. My favorite dinner is fish tacos with lots of cilantro – just make sure to grill the fish, don't fry it!

Cilantro Soap

And yes, I realize that when it comes to cilantro, people either love it or hate it. If you think cilantro tastes a little like soap, there's a solid scientific reason: your "cilantro taste" is genetic. It turns out that people who hate the herb share certain genes that smell "aldehyde chemicals," substances found in both cilantro and – you guessed it – soap. So you're not being picky; you inherited it!

But even though coriander and cilantro come from the same plant, they don't taste anything alike. If you're not a fan of cilantro, give the dried form, coriander, a chance. It has a nutty, slightly sweet taste – it might remind you of cinnamon. You probably already eat more coriander than you realize; it's used for flavoring cookies, pastries, cheese, sausage and processed meats like hot dogs and lunchmeat (although I certainly don't recommend consuming pastries and hot dogs to get your daily dose of coriander.)

There are plenty of easy ways to use dried coriander in powder form. It pairs well with curry and cumin so you can add it to spice rubs, sauces, chilis, and soups. . The spice tastes great with carrots, so try sprinkling a little on top of a carrot salad or stir some into carrot soup. It works well in pumpkin soup, too. (For a bonus health boost with that soup, add a little dried ginger!)

A Seven-Way Tie for the #10 Spice!

These seven spices might be a little less familiar than the headliners, or maybe there hasn't been as much research on them (yet). But they still deliver healthy perks big-time! They deserve a strong supporting role in your diet, and I encourage you to start eating them.

Cardamom – the diet protector

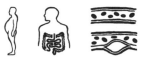

This one is royalty, nicknamed the "Queen of Spices" (black pepper is the "King") because it was a favorite of the elite, and because its flavor is almost feminine compared to other spices – floral, lemony, with a hint of mint. That might be why it was once considered an aphrodisiac. Its health advantages ran the gamut; people used it to remedy inflamed eyelids, tooth and gum infections, lung congestion, sore throat, and more serious afflictions like gallstones, kidney disease, stomach disorders and tuberculosis, as well as an antidote for poison and snakebites.

The benefits we see today are broad, too, but relevant because Americans eat so poorly. In essence, cardamom may help counter the effects of our bad diets, especially when we tend to eat too many carbohydrates. One study showed that subjects who ate cardamom gained less extra weight (and, importantly, less belly fat) and avoided increases in their blood sugar, cholesterol and inflammation levels.

Cardamom also helps relax the gut to help improve digestion and may improve heart health by lowering blood pressure and preventing blood clots according to animal and test tube studies.

Fenugreek – the lesser known blood sugar hero

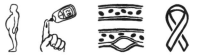

If you even know what this spice is, you're a step ahead of most people. It's a plant related to peas, which is more obvious when you see its round, yellow seeds. Fenugreek is popular in the Mediterranean region; people sometimes roast the seeds, grind them and dissolve the powder in a tea, though the leaves are edible, too.

Also called "Greek hay," fenugreek was used centuries ago to induce childbirth and help soothe burns. The Greeks also believed it cured infections, while the Romans used it to remedy breathing and stomach problems, fevers and wounds. Because of the seeds' vivid color, it also was used to dye wool.

For the past 30 years, scientists have studied fenugreek's ability to control blood sugar levels, and they're fairly certain that it plays a positive role: a review of 10 studies found that fenugreek not only lowered blood sugar, it went on to help with long-term glucose levels. That effect was seen most strongly in people already diagnosed with type 2 diabetes. According to scientists at John Hopkins University, fenugreek is also a potent anti-cancer agent. It also reduces cholesterol, and animal studies have found that it may help reduce fatty liver disease, cataracts, gallstones, and kidney stones, making it an all- around all-star.

I often use a supplement containing fenugreek with patients to control blood sugar, but I admit I haven't cooked with it a lot. But my pal, author and ultramarathon runner Dean Karnazes loves it, and he generously gave me a great fenugreek-containing recipe you can find later in the book. I definitely encourage you to give this lesser known spice a try - the seeds should be cooked or ground before use and be sure to add it sparingly at first to avoid overpowering your cooking.

Sage – a wise choice for many reasons

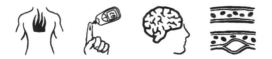

Sage is another blood sugar and cholesterol champion, though several thousand years ago the Greeks and Romans used it to preserve meat, and Arab physicians thought it could boost our chances of immortality. Native Americans made "smudge sticks," small bundles of sage that they burned in energy-clearing ceremonies. That use continues today; if you engage a feng shui practitioner to enhance the energy in your home, for instance, that person is likely to burn a smudge stick to clear negative energy from the space.

Today we know sage reduces blood sugar and cholesterol levels. Researchers recently studied a group of individuals with type 2 diabetes and high cholesterol who also were taking medication to lower those levels. They found that when they added sage to people's daily routine, it reduced their blood sugar and LDL (bad) cholesterol, and increased their HDL (good) cholesterol, even more than taking meds alone. A bonus benefit: sage contains one of the same anti-inflammatory compounds as oregano, rosemary and thyme.

Sage is also a powerhouse for brain health. Several human studies have found that a sage extract led to faster recall, improved mood, and less age-related memory loss. In addition, an Iranian study found that it may improve brain function in people with mild to moderate Alzheimer's disease.

The flavor of sage can be intense, so when you cook with it, a little goes a long way. If you buy it fresh, it makes a nice chicken marinade along with lemon juice, lemon zest and garlic. Italian cooks chop it, mix it with melted butter and stir it into pasta. Dried sage is good in a pork rub, but it's compatible with any meat or poultry.

Saffron – the mood booster

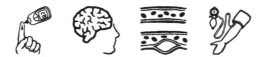

Saffron's vivid orange color and grassy, sweet taste have made it one of the priciest spices throughout history. It's still used in making perfumes and dyes, and in religious ceremonies in some countries.

Middle Eastern healers have treated eye disorders, earaches, toothaches, headaches, ulcers, wounds, urinary problems and women's issues with saffron. In modern times, a number of studies have shown it reduces blood cholesterol and sugar levels, and lowers blood pressure. It might even help keeps us from gaining weight: one study showed it was just as effective for losing weight as a weight-loss medication.

One of the most remarkable benefits of this colorful spice is its ability to improve symptoms of mild to moderate depression. Numerous studies have found saffron extract to be as effective as commonly used anti-depressant medications and to be far more effective than placebo. In addition, saffron may ease several of the symptoms of PMS, especially menstrual cramps, and may also help with anxiety and insomnia.

And one of its active ingredients, crocin, increases blood flow to the retina which may decrease age-related macular degeneration, the leading cause of blindness in the United States.

I'm a big fan of Rumi Spice, a company started by a group of U.S. military veterans who partnered with Afghan farmers to produce a red gold saffron that is not only a chef favorite, it has had a profound impact on the community and employs 75 Afghan women. For more information about this amazing company go to www.rumispice.com and check out the delicious saffron recipe later in this book provided by Rumi's CEO, Kimberly Jung.

She also made these 5 suggestions for incorporating more saffron into your diet:

1. Drink it simply, as a tea. Saffron has a distinct, ethereal flavor that is enjoyed by many on its own. Steep a pinch (6-8 threads) in a cup of hot water and watch it turn a bright, golden color.
2. Infuse it in rice or risotto. Saffron dissolves easily, so it does well in soups, as well as rice dishes with plenty of H2O and time to infuse. A traditional Milanese dish consists of just saffron, risotto, white wine, and butter.

3. Steep a pinch of saffron in warm water for 20 minutes and you can incorporate that "saffron concentrate" into any sauce of your choice.
4. For baked goods such as bread, cookies or Rice Krispies™ treats, turn to your mortar and pestle to grind saffron into a powder and incorporate directly into the dough or mix.
5. To quickly bring out the flavor and balance it with a creamy medium like yogurt, steep saffron threads in fresh lemon juice. The acidity brings out the flavor of saffron very well.

Tarragon – the French connection for insulin resistance

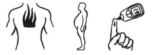

We believe tarragon originally came from Siberia and Central Asia, but during the Crusades it made its way across Europe. Over time it was used to treat snake bites, dog bites, toothaches, insomnia and even bad breath. St. Catherine, returning from a visit with Pope Clement VI, helped tarragon's migration when she brought the spice home to France.

In addition to fighting inflammation, research shows that tarragon might help prevent diabetes in those at high risk.. One group of people diagnosed with pre-diabetes took tarragon supplements for three months, and by the end of the study they showed better long term control over their blood sugar and better sensitivity to insulin.

Tarragon is a favorite ingredient in French cooking, especially in a béarnaise sauce or in chicken, fish or vegetable dishes. But if you don't feel like cooking an elaborate supper, just chop (or tear up) some tarragon and mix it with greens in a salad, or sprinkle it over pasta or rice, just as you would parsley.

Nutmeg – an anti-aging secret weapon

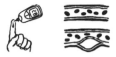

Nutmeg is in everyone's cupboard now, but centuries ago it was so expensive and rare that wars were fought in Europe to gain control of its production. In the Arab world it was believed to be an aphrodisiac and a cure for stomach ailments, while in Indian Vedic medicine it was given to people with headaches, fever and bad breath. In Europe it was even believed to ward off the Plague.

Modern research finds that the active components in nutmeg not only improve blood sugar levels, they also may help curtail weight gain and reduce cholesterol. In one study of mice, researchers saw that even with a high-fat diet, adding one of nutmeg's active ingredients resulted in lower body weight, blood sugar levels and cholesterol levels, compared to just eating high-fat foods.

Nutmeg may also help keep you looking younger. A study in South Korea found that it helped support a protein that maintains the elasticity of your skin, which can lead to tighter, more youthful skin. In addition, like rosemary, it protects the skin from the damaging effects of UV radiation which can decrease your risk of wrinkles, sun spots, and skin cancer.

If you use pumpkin spice (sometimes called "pumpkin pie spice") in your baking, you're already using nutmeg because it's a key ingredient – but it's not only used in desserts. You can find ground, dried nutmeg in any grocery; it tastes great sprinkled on vegetables like sweet potatoes, butternut squash, carrots and cabbage. It's tasty sprinkled on fruit, too, such as bananas, pears, mangoes, or fresh or baked apples. Use it at breakfast on quiches, eggs or French toast, and you can dress up your hot tea, cocoa, coffee or eggnog with a little nutmeg, and get its super health benefits at the same time.

Basil – the stress solution

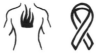

Did someone say pesto? I'm there! Basil is the main ingredient in one of the most luscious sauces ever invented – and fortunately, it has great health benefits as well.

Traditionally thought of as part of Italian cooking, it is actually native to India where it is believed to have been in use for 5000 years. Basil is known as the "king of herbs" or the "royal herb" and to the Italians, basil is a symbol of love. The ancient Egyptians and ancient Greeks held the belief that basil would open the gates of heaven for a person passing on. In India, they put basil in the mouth of the dying to ensure they reached God. In Europe, basil is set in the hands of the dead to ensure a safe journey.

In Ayurvedic medicine, basil was used to treat headaches, colds, stomach problems, malaria, poisoning, inflammation, heart disease, and even snake bites.

Basil is a powerful inflammation fighter – and from what you've already read, you know that lowering inflammation means reducing pain and decreasing your risk of a host of other diseases including heart disease, diabetes, dementia, and cancer. It is also a potent anti-oxidant which may also help protect you from cancer and heart disease.

In addition, basil may play an important role in stress reduction, something that most of us could use these days. Several animal studies have found that the active ingredients in basil reduce levels of the stress hormone cortisol and soothed overactive adrenal glands (where cortisol is produced). It may also reduce the formation of ulcers associated with stress.

If you're thinking of growing your own food, basil is a good place to start because it's easy to grow. And if you make your own pesto with it (and who wouldn't?), you may find that you can cut the amount of olive oil significantly because the basil itself is so delicious, it doesn't need as much fat as most recipes call for.

One of the best things about basil is that you can use it so casually – no measuring needed. Tear up a handful and top your homemade pizza with it (use whole wheat crust, just a little cheese and lots of herbs it the pizza sauce). Toss whole leaves in a salad with other greens or use it instead of lettuce on a turkey sandwich. Make a quick pasta dressing with fresh chopped basil, olive oil, lemon juice. Or, purée basil with olive oil and lemon juice and drizzle the sauce over salmon. Delicious!

One last honorable mention…

Dill – a cholesterol champion

I ran out of time and space but no book of spices would be complete without including dill. It's a wonderfully flavorful herb with a 5000 year history of medicinal use and several research papers show its benefit in reducing cholesterol. It is delicious as part of a dip or can be added to soups and rice dishes.

Here is an easy-to-read chart of spices and their potential health benefits. Simply find the spice you plan on using and read across to see all the various health benefits that spice has to offer. Notice that all the spices have numerous benefits.

For optimal health, I recommend consuming a variety of spices, or you may to choose focus on specific spices based on your health concerns.

AT-A-GLANCE SPICE CHART

	Inflammation	Belly fat/insulin resistance	Diabetes	Arthritis	Brain health	Gut health	High cholesterol	High blood pressure	Cancer	Metabolism booster
Cinnamon	✓	✓	✓		✓		✓	✓		
Turmeric	✓	✓	✓	✓	✓	✓			✓	
Cayenne	✓	✓				✓			✓	✓
Ginger	✓	✓		✓		✓			✓	
Rosemary	✓			✓	✓		✓		✓	
Oregano	✓					✓			✓	
Cumin	✓	✓				✓	✓			
Thyme	✓				✓	✓			✓	
Coriander/ Cilantro	✓		✓			✓	✓			
Cardamom		✓				✓		✓		
Fenugreek		✓	✓				✓		✓	
Sage	✓		✓		✓	✓	✓			
Saffron			✓		✓		✓	✓		
Tarragon	✓	✓	✓							
Nutmeg			✓				✓			
Basil	✓								✓	

SPICE BLENDS, TRIOS, AND TIPS

A fun way to eat more spices – and be rewarded with more of their tremendous health bonuses – is to use spice blends in your cooking. I've listed six of my favorite blends below, with their ingredients and popular uses. You've already read why the spices in these blends make you healthier; now we can think about combining them, cooking and eating delicious, spicy, health-boosting meals!

As you'll see, there are variations for most blends. There's no wrong way to concoct them – there are plenty of options here; truly, you can add a little of this, a little of that, whatever tastes best to you. At the end of this section I've provided some tips on buying and storing spices, because we all need a refresher course in that.

Chili Powder

Like all spice blends, everyone who makes chili powder has their own recipe. They usually start with ancho chiles, paprika, cumin and Mexican oregano. Some people add salt, garlic powder, cayenne powder, coriander, ground black pepper and onion powder to the mix. You might use more than one type of chili pepper; you can choose from Aleppo, chipotle, chile de arbol, Cheongyang, jalapeño,

New Mexico, pasilla and piri piri chili peppers.

The two words that best describe chili powder are spicy and smoky. Sprinkle it on pork, beef, chicken, fish and stews; it's also good for adding zest to vegetables – sweet potatoes, squash, corn, cauliflower, tomato and almost any kind of beans. I also add it to soups, sauces, dips, salad dressings, dry rubs and marinades.

Herbs de Provence

This romantic blend is named for one of the world's great romantic places, probably because Provence is the home of lavender, one of the popular (but not required) ingredients in the blend. Rosemary, marjoram, thyme, tarragon, sage and oregano are the basics; dried lavender flowers are often added, along with orange zest, fennel seed, dried basil, dried Italian parsley, bay powder or bay leaf, savory (a relative of rosemary and thyme), chervil and mint.

Herbs de Provence has a woodsy, fresh, fragrant, floral aroma and flavor. If you prefer a more smoky blend you can omit the lavender, orange and mint. But I adore that combination; I can almost taste the French countryside when I eat it.

Use Herbs de Provence on grilled foods, pork, beef, lamb, stews and fish, as well as cheese, potatoes, squash, zucchini, tomatoes, eggplant and onions. It also can add a different tone to pizza sauce, popcorn topping, soups, marinades, dry rubs and salad dressings. My easiest way to use herbs de Provence is to mix it into a good-quality olive oil and use it summer grilling.

Curry Powder

Nothing else tastes like a good curry powder. It's made of turmeric, coriander, cumin, fenugreek and red pepper. There are plenty of variations; you can choose from cloves, garlic, cinnamon, cardamom, ginger, black pepper, caraway, mustard seed, nutmeg, curry leaf, chili peppers and fennel.

Curry is a distinct, warm, spicy, strong flavor. Depending on the cuisine, it's added to lentils, chicken, pork, beef and tofu; or vegetable dishes like pumpkin, cauliflower, broccoli, zucchini, squash, cabbage, onions and green beans. Curry can flavor your main dish or a side; add it to stir fries, curries, rice, marinades, sauces and soups.

Cajun Seasoning

The base ingredients in Cajun seasoning are black pepper, cayenne pepper, cumin, paprika and thyme. Some producers add salt, garlic powder, onion powder and oregano. (Shopper alert: a lot of commercial Cajun seasonings contain way too much salt for me. If you don't like food that tastes over-salty, ask your grocer which brands contain less.)

Whatever the variation, Cajun seasoning usually is hot, spicy and peppery tasting. Use it on blackened fish, shellfish, chicken, turkey, beef, pork and sausage. You also can add it to vegetables, including onions, bell peppers, carrots, celery, and potatoes. It works in rice, gumbo, dry rubs and creamy sauces for dips or pasta.

Chinese Five Spice

This is a less familiar spice blend to home cooks, but if you like Chinese food, jump in and try it. The main ingredients are cinnamon, cloves, fennel, star anise and Szechuan peppercorns; variations include ginger, nutmeg, cardamom, licorice, galangal, cumin, turmeric and mandarin orange peel.

Obviously, it usually has more than five ingredients. But the blend is called Chinese Five Spice because it gives you the five flavors of sweet, sour, bitter, pungent and salty. Some describe it as tasting "warm." Use this blend on pork, duck, goose, beef, tofu and fish. It's good on vegetables, too: shiitake mushrooms, broccoli, cauliflower, bell peppers, zucchini, carrots, onions and celery. Add it to stir fries, rice, marinades and dry rubs.

Italian Blend

You know these ingredients; they even sound like an Italian dish: oregano, thyme, rosemary, basil and marjoram, with garlic powder, crushed red pepper flakes, sage and cilantro for variation.

Italian blend gives off an earthy, sweet, fresh and peppery taste. It pairs easily with chicken, fish, beef, pork, cheese and tofu, or, if you're making a vegetable dish, add it to tomatoes, potatoes, eggplant, zucchini and squash.

You've probably eaten it in Italian dishes: pasta, pizza sauce or with olive oil as a bread dip. But it's also good in salad dressing, stuffing, soups, stews, dry rubs and marinades.

Spice Breakfast Trios

Smoothies – You can use either protein powder (aim for 14-21 g protein per serving with limited added sugar) or Greek yogurt (3/4 cup – 1 cup plain low-fat or non-fat) to add protein to any of these smoothie combinations. Feel free to mix and match fresh or frozen fruit, spices and healthy fats and add leafy green vegetables to boost nutrients even more and use stevia to taste.

Fruit	Spice	Healthy Fat
½ banana or 1 cup of cherries	¼ - ½ tsp cinnamon	1-2 tbsp almond butter
1 cup strawberries	1-2 tbsp fresh basil, thyme or rosemary	1-2 tbsp chia seeds
1 cup peaches	¼ - ½ tsp ginger	2 tbsp flaxseeds
1 small apple or pear, diced	¼ - ½ tsp cinnamon or allspice	1-2 tbsp peanut butter
1 small pear, diced	¼ - ½ tsp ginger	1-2 tbsp almond butter
½ mango, diced or 1 cup	¼ tsp ginger or 1-2 tbsp fresh mint or basil	¼ avocado
½ banana	¼ tsp turmeric	2 tbsp walnuts
1 cup blueberry or blackberry	1-2 tbsp fresh mint or sage	1-2 tbsp chia seeds

Fresh herbs work great in smoothies but if you only have dried on hand cut amount used by half. Add ice to smoothies to taste and thickness desired (I like mine pretty thick so I drink it more slowly!) In addition, these combinations work great for **yogurt parfaits**.

Scrambles are also a great way to start your day with spices. Here are some fun combination including a little cheese (which is completely optional) for added flavor and to keep you fuller longer. I recommend using 1 egg plus 2-3 whites or ½ cup of egg substitute per serving and cooking vegetables almost fully before adding the egg mix. Then just top with cheese at the end. Again, feel free to mix and match spices, vegetables and cheeses or bake these in muffin cups or a big frittata and heat and eat all week. Feel free to add a little salt and pepper to taste and use non-stick cooking spray.

Vegetables	Spices	Cheese (optional)
½ cup diced green peppers + ¼ cup diced onions	1/8 tsp turmeric + pinch black pepper	2 tbsp mozzarella
1 cup spinach + ½ cup sliced mushrooms	1 tbsp fresh or 1-2 tsp thyme	2 tbsp crumbled goat cheese
½ cup diced zucchini + ½ cup diced tomatoes	1-2 tbsp fresh rosemary or 1-2 tsp. dried	1-2 tbsp fresh parmesan
1/3 cup black beans + ¼ cup salsa	1/8 tsp cumin + 1/8 tsp chili powder	1-2 tbsp shredded cheddar or Mexican style shredded cheese

Buying Spices

You can buy spices at your local supermarket, natural co-op, farmers market, ethnic markets (Indian, Asian, Mexican), specialty stores or online. If you're ambitious, you can grow spices fresh in your garden or on the windowsill.

Tips for Storing Spices

The best general rule is, to keep your dried spices fresh, keep them away from light, heat, moisture and air. It's best to store them in a dry, cool, dark place such as a cabinet or pantry.

More Spice Storage Tips

Whether they're fresh, canned or in a jar, keep spices away from the stove, furnace vents, microwave, sunlight, windows, coffee maker, kettle, sink, dishwasher and the countertop.

Ground spices will keep for one year, while whole spices (such as peppercorns) will keep for two to three years.

Fresh herbs will keep anywhere from a few days to several weeks. Fresh basil and cilantro can be stored in a container of water on the kitchen counter after you've trimmed the ends, like a bouquet of flowers.

For fresh thyme and rosemary, loosely wrap them in plastic wrap and place them in the warmest part of the refrigerator, such as a compartment on the door. You can add a crumpled paper towel as a safeguard against moisture. Do not rinse the herbs until you're ready to use them.

To store fresh oregano, wrap it in a damp paper towel and place it in a plastic bag in the refrigerator.

Fresh turmeric can be stored in the refrigerator or a cool dry place; it will keep for up to three weeks.

Refrigerate fresh ginger root in a plastic bag. It will keep fresh for two to three weeks.

SEVEN WAYS TO SLIM DOWN WITH SPICES

This is not a diet book, but the potential slimming power of spices is impressive and research continues to reveal their benefits in terms of both weight loss and disease prevention. While the effect of individual spices on weight loss, in most cases, are subtle, their cumulative effect on weight loss, weight maintenance and improved health could be significant, so including them both frequently and consistently in your diet is an essential component of any successful weight loss and healthy lifestyle plan.

Here are 7 ways that spices can help you slim down

Spices fight inflammation. Spices including turmeric, basil, ginger, sage, saffron, oregano, coriander, cumin, nutmeg, oregano, thyme, chili peppers (cayenne, paprika, red pepper, chili powder), rosemary and garlic can help your body fight inflammation by up-regulating or increasing anti-inflammatory genes and proteins and down-regulating or decreasing pro inflammatory genes and proteins. An anti-inflammatory diet is associated with improved weight loss and less weight gain over time as well as a decreased risk of diabetes, heart disease, cancer and dementia. Green tea, which is from leaves and therefore closely related to herbs, contains a powerful compound, EGCG, which can also help fight inflammation.

Spices improve your body's response to insulin and improve blood sugar control. By decreasing inflammation, spices improve your body's response to insulin, but several spices including turmeric, fenugreek, ginger, nutmeg, sage, thyme, cinnamon, curry leaf and chili pepper (cayenne, paprika, red pepper, chili powder) have a more direct effect on blood sugar regulation. They help decrease blood sugar levels, improve your body's response to insulin, and decrease your body's resistance to insulin so you need less insulin to do the same job. Reducing insulin levels is important as too much insulin can lead to excess fat storage, especially the inflammatory fat stored deeper in the belly region (also known as visceral fat). Green tea EGCG may also help with insulin response and reducing belly fat.

Spices increase the breakdown of fat (lipolysis), the use of fat for fuel (fat oxidation), and decreases fat accumulation in fat cells (lipogenesis). Spices including turmeric, cumin, rosemary, nutmeg, sage, and cayenne pepper are beneficial in this respect through their action on hormones and proteins involved in lipolysis and fat oxidation and cumin, turmeric, ginger, drumstick leaf, curry leaf and cayenne pepper have been shown in clinical studies to directly help with weight loss. Chemicals in green tea (EGCG) also help increase fat oxidation.

Spices function as prebiotics. A recent study by my colleagues at UCLA Center for Human Nutrition found that spices including black pepper, cayenne pepper, cinnamon, ginger, oregano, rosemary and turmeric have a pre-biotic effect, supporting the growth of good bacteria (Lactobacillus and Bifidobaterium species) in your gut. Emerging science suggests an important role of the bacteria in your gut (known as the microbiome) in obesity, inflammation, and insulin resistance in addition to their important role in digestion.

Spices can help you feel fuller faster. Capsaicin, one of the active ingredients in Chili pepper (cayenne especially), can help reduce appetite. How it does this is not completely understood but it is likely due to stimulation of a specific receptor in your digestive track associated with satiety (fullness). Research shows that ginger may also reduce hunger, and prebiotics (which include the spices listed above) help increase gut hormones (GLP-1, PYY) which can help control appetite. Two studies of fenugreek have shown that it also increases satiety (fullness) and can lead to decreased caloric intake. Green tea EGCG has also been shown to reduce hunger, especially when reducing calories.

Spices increase your metabolism. Capsaicin, a chemical found in Chili pepper (especially cayenne), can increase the number of calories your burn daily by approximately 5 percent, a modest effect which can really add up over time. Ginger can also modestly increase the thermic effect of food (the calories you burn digesting, absorbing and processing food) which can also be beneficial over time.

Spices improve the flavor of food without adding calories or sodium (like fat and salt do). This is true for all spices. In order to stick with a diet (i.e. way of eating) long term, food has to taste good, and spices are one of the best (and easiest) ways to make food taste great without adding excess fat, sugar, and salt.

Slimming Spice Lifestyle Overview

This is a nutrition guide, not a diet book. As a nutrition MD and weight loss expert for the last 17 years, I didn't want to write another diet book because *there is no one size fits all when it comes to weight loss.* There are so many different ways to lose weight, and much of my approach with patients is very personalized and depends on their genes, lifestyle, culture, medical history, and food preferences. The goal of this book is to get you excited about spices because they are a super healthy addition to any diet (from paleo to vegan and everything in between), and they may help you lose weight more easily along with a healthy lifestyle.

I will give you some basic direction but feel free to follow any diet plan that you enjoy and that can stick with. Whatever diet plan you choose, just make sure to add lots of spices.

Despite what some popular diet plans claim, to lose weight you do have to reduce calories, but just as importantly, you need to optimize the quality of your calories (and it helps to burn more calories too). Here are some of the most important diet, exercise and behavior principles based on my 17 years of experience helping patients lose weight and improve their health.

General Weight Loss Recommendations

Before getting started, measure your waist – if you are a woman and your waist is greater than 35 inches or a man with a waist greater than 40 inches, you will most likely lose more weight in the short term if you cut back on grains (pasta, rice, crackers, bread, cereal) and starchy carbohydrates like potatoes, corn, beans and peas. Limit yourself to a maximum of 2 servings per day (about 1/2 cup, 1 slice, or 15 g of carbs). For best results, replace starchy carbs with healthy fat (nuts, seeds, healthy oils, avocado). I also recommend limiting your fruit to no more than 2 servings per day. If your waist does not exceed these guidelines, you can choose to limit fat or carbohydrates to reduce your calories and you can have up to 3 servings of fruit per day.

Below are 7 basic tips to get you started

1. Make most of your grains are **whole grains**.
2. Eat at least **5 servings** of non-starchy **vegetables** per day (1 serving = ½ cup cooked, 1 cup raw)
3. **Limit added sugar** (especially if you fall into the large waist group)
4. Consume **lean protein** (chicken, fish, turkey, lean red meat, protein powder, low fat dairy, eggs/egg whites) with every meal and most snacks to control hunger, keep blood sugar stable and preserve muscle. I generally recommend about 2-3 ounces at breakfast, 3-5 ounces at lunch, 4-6 ounces at dinner, and 1-2 ounces per snack (1 ounce = 7 grams). If you are smaller, less active, and a female eat towards the lower end of the recommendations.
5. **Watch your serving size of fats**, even the healthy ones. This is one of the biggest mistakes that I see in my office, especially for women. Pay attention to serving sizes even if you are reducing carbohydrates. Here are some common fat serving sizes:
    - 1 tbsp. oil = 3 fats
    - 1 tsp. oil or butter = 1 fat
    - ¼ small avocado = 1 fat
    - 2 tbsp. seeds = 1 fat
    - ¼ cup nuts = 2 fats
6. **Exercise is essential** for long term weight loss. Aim for at least 150 minutes or cardio and 2 days of strength training per week. I'm a big fan of high intensity interval training (HIIT) a once or twice a week to give your metabolism and weight loss an extra boost. There are lots of different HIIT programs so go online or to the app store and find one that works for you. Whatever exercise program you start, make

sure that it is something you enjoy and will continue so that the weight loss lasts.

7. **Build better eating behavior**. This is also essential for optimal weight loss. My top 3 suggestions are:

- Always have a plan and/or be prepared
- Control your eating environment by building in portion control by eating off smaller plates and bowls and keeping less healthy foods out of sight (higher in the cabinet or at the back of the freezer)
- Manage stress as much as possible (I know, its easier said than done but consider yoga, meditation (an app is ok), socializing with friends, or just taking a break for a cup of tea. Trust me, it makes a difference when it comes to weight loss!

I realize that this is not a very specific diet plan, but I'm confident that this is more than enough to get you started and again, the main goal of this book is to get you to spice up your diet.

SPICE UP, SLIM DOWN RECIPES

The recipe section of this book is divided into two parts – in the first part, I worked with professional chefs Sandra Mallut and Aaron Robbins to develop some fabulous, spice-filled recipes, many of which are very versatile and not too challenging (I actually made many of these to test them).

In the second part of the recipe section, I reached out to several dozen of my celebrity friends, trainers, athletes, doctors and health experts to get their favorite spice-rich recipes. Many of them have also written books so they generously let me share their wonderful recipes with you. As you will see, a few are celebrity chefs, but most are not, and many are busy parents like me who are just trying to do their best to stay healthy and keep their families happy and healthy.

Dressings, Dips, Sauces, and Appetizers

Tomato Basil Dijon Vinaigrette
Yields ½ cup

Ingredients

2 tbsp dried basil or fresh basil chopped
2 tbsp balsamic vinegar
1 tbsp chopped red onion
1 tsp Dijon mustard

10 cherry or grape tomatoes or chopped tomatoes or about 2 oz
¾ tsp chopped garlic
2 tbsp olive oil
Pinch Kosher Salt
Pinch Black Pepper

Directions

Put basil, vinegar, onions, mustard, tomatoes and garlic in food processor or blender and process until smooth. With processor or blender on add the olive oil and process until combined then it is ready. Taste and then season with salt and pepper. Store in air tight container and can be stored in cooler for up to 3 days. Best to bring to room temp when serving.

Variations

Add different fresh herbs, other kinds of mustard, different tomatoes from green to yellow, spices you can add red pepper flakes for a bit of heat.

Basic Red Sauce

Ingredients

3 tbsp olive oil
2 tbsp chopped garlic
2 tbsp minced onion
1 can (28oz) crushed tomatoes
1 can (28oz) tomato puree
3 tbsp. dried basil, oregano, rosemary – 1 tbsp of each
½ tsp cayenne
½ tsp black pepper
½ tsp kosher salt

Directions

First heat oil in a large saucepan over medium heat and sautee garlic and onion until tender stir in crushed tomatoes, tomato puree, cayenne, salt, pepper, and Italian seasonings. Now reduce heat to low and simmer for at least 40 minutes. This sauce can be stored in refrigerator for up to a week and frozen for up to 3 – 4 weeks.

Basic Yogurt Dip
Yields 2 cups

Ingredients

1 cup plain Greek-style or plain yogurt
1/2 cucumber, roughly chopped
Juice of 1/2 lemon and top with some lemon zest
2 tbsp fresh herbs (any combination of dill, mint, cilantro, and basil)
1 tbsp extra virgin olive oil
1 clove garlic, minced
1 tsp cumin
1/2 tsp coriander
¼ tsp kosher salt

Directions

Medium bowl combine all ingredients and then let sit for at least 30 minutes for the flavors to meld and serve. Can also be stored in cooler for couple days.

Variations:
Change out the fresh herbs or add some heat with red pepper flakes, paprika or cayenne pepper

Nectarine Relish
Yields 4 cups

Ingredients

3 ripe nectarines, chopped
1 cup chopped cherry tomatoes
¼ cup red onion, chopped
¾ cup corn if frozen thaw first
2 tsp Italian parsley or mint, chopped
1/2 tsp cumin - optional
½ tsp red pepper flakes
1 tbsp olive oil
Pinch Kosher Salt
Pinch Black Pepper

Directions

Combine all ingredients and serve. Can be refrigerated and used for several days. Great on a taco salad or with fish or chicken tacos.

Variations
Fruit can be changed out peaches, plums, apples and fresh herbs can be changed out to taste

Herb Parmesan Crisp
Makes 16 crisps 20 calories/crisp

Ingredients

1 cup Shredded Parmigiano/Reggiano
1-2 tbsp dried herb of your choice (I love thyme; if you like a little spicy kick use a few flakes of crushed red pepper)
non-stick cooking spray

Directions

Lightly spray baking sheet with oil. Using a tablespoon, place Parmesan/Reggiano in mounds approximately 2 inches apart on baking sheet.
Sprinkle each mound with a pinch of thyme, a few flakes of crushed red pepper, or the seasoning of your choice.
Bake at 350 degrees for 8 minutes or until golden brown. Cool completely before removing from baking sheet.

Entrees

Spicy Fish Tacos
Yields 4 – 6 tacos

Ingredients

2 tilapia fish fillets
2 scallions, chopped
2 garlic cloves, minced
1 avocado, chopped
1 cup black beans, drained of liquid
½ cup canned or cooked corn, drained
2 tbsp olive oil
1 tbsp cumin
1 tsp chili powder
¼ - ½ tsp cayenne pepper
Package of small corn tortillas
Finish with lemon or lime juice, salt, pepper
Optional: salsa, pico de gallo, fresh cilantro (shredded)

Directions

Combine the chili powder, cayenne, and cumin then coat the tilapia (both sides).
Heat the olive oil (can use the chili pepper oil) in a pan over medium heat, then cook the tilapia for 3 minutes per side. Remove from heat and chop or shred the fish fillets.
Add the scallions and garlic to the pan and sauté 30 seconds to 1

minute.

Add corn to the pan and stir, cooking the corn until it's slightly blackened.

Add the beans and cook 1 to 2 minutes then remove the pan from the heat

Warm tortillas and spoon the corn and bean mix into a soft taco tortilla, then top with tilapia and chopped avocado. Add your favorite salsa or pico de gallo, salsa, lemon or lime juice, cilantro, salt, and/or pepper to taste.

Spice Rubbed Grilled Chicken Dinner
4 servings

Ingredients

4 chicken breasts without skin
1 tbsp cumin
1 tsp curry powder
½ tsp ground ginger
½ tsp kosher salt
⅛ tsp cayenne pepper
1 tbsp olive oil

Directions

Mix all ingredients together and rubbed all over chicken and then grill on the grill or in your grill pan on the stove – you can get grill marks and then finish off in oven and do a brush with olive oil mid-way through to keep chicken moist and cook chicken to internal temperature of 165 for food safety.

Complete meal option: Cut chicken into bite size pieces. Coat wok with olive oil or non-stick cooking spray and cook chicken for 2 minutes. Add 2-4 cups of broccoli and 2 cups of sliced mushrooms and seasoning blend and stir fry until vegetables tender and chicken bite are fully cooked – approximately 8-10 minutes.

Salmon Spice or Herb Kebabs
4 servings

Ingredients

1 pound boneless, skinless wild salmon fillet, cut into chunks
1-2 zucchinis, sliced into thick rounds
1 large red onion, cut into chunks
½ teaspoon fine sea salt
1-2 tsp garlic, chopped
1 tablespoon finely chopped fresh rosemary or dry rosemary or Spice
Cumin or Cilantro
¼ cup extra-virgin olive oil
3 tbsp lime juice – one lime cut in quarters to finish
½ tsp ground black pepper

Directions

Place salmon, zucchini, and onion in a shallow baking dish or large
zip lock bag and sprinkle with salt and pepper. Whisk together garlic,
rosemary, oil and lime juice in a small bowl. Pour mixture over
salmon and vegetables, toss and marinate 15 to 30 minutes.

Prepare a grill (or broiler) for medium-high heat. Skewer salmon and
vegetables, (If using wooden skewers, soak in water for 30 minutes
before assembling.) Grill kebabs, turning once and glaze with any
leftover marinade until salmon is cooked through and vegetables are
tender, about 7 to 9 minutes. Squeeze lime juice over kebab before
serving.

Mustard Spiced Salmon Filets
4 servings

Ingredients

2 teaspoons whole-grain mustard or your favorite
1 tsp honey (optional)
¼ tsp ground turmeric

¼ tsp ground red pepper
1/8 tsp garlic powder
¼ tsp kosher salt
4 (6-ounce) salmon fillets

Directions

Preheat your oven broiler. Combine first 6 ingredients in a small bowl, stirring well with a fork or whisk and then rub mustard mixture evenly over each fillet (not skin side) (use paper towel to wipe any moisture off skin of fish to get the best crispy skin), add filets to pan that has been prepared with cooking spray skin side down.
Broil 8 minutes or until fish flakes easily when tested with a fork or until desired degree of doneness.

Spiced Quinoa
4 servings

Ingredients

1 cup rinsed and drained quinoa
1 tsp ground ginger
1 tsp ground cumin
1 tsp ground coriander
1 tsp ground turmeric
2 tbsp vegetable or olive oil
2 cups boiling water
Salt and pepper to taste
Vegetables (optional) add your favorite chopped vegetable to this dish

Directions

Get your water boiling while you get the rest of the recipe moving forward. Using a larger sized saucepan brown spices in oil then add quinoa (rinse first) and stir well. Add boiling water; simmer until water is absorbed. Option: Serve with a low sodium soy sauce or fish sauce to give a tang.

My Mom's Spicy Turkey Chili
Approximately 6 servings

Ingredients

1 pound lean ground turkey
1 (28 ounce) can petite diced tomatoes
1 (16 ounce) can pinto beans, rinsed and drained
2 teaspoons chili powder
½ teaspoon ground cumin
½ teaspoon ground cayenne pepper
¼ teaspoon ground black pepper
¼ teaspoon salt

Directions

Spray a large pot or skillet with spray cooking oil. Brown turkey and drain off any fat. Add chili powder, cayenne pepper, cumin, salt and pepper to turkey and continue to cook for several minutes while stirring constantly. Add diced tomatoes and pinto beans to seasoned turkey and bring to a boil. Reduce heat to simmer and cook for 20 minutes, stirring occasionally. To make chili thinner add ½ cup of water while simmering. (serve with a dab of low fat sour cream…but don't tell Melina!)

Soups and Sides

Spiced Sweet Potato Bisque
6-8 servings

Ingredients

5lbs sweet potatoes, peeled and large dice
1.5 cup shallots, sliced
2 tbsp garlic, chopped
1 cup almond milk
7cups vegetable stock
¼ tsp ground clove
¼ tsp cayenne pepper

½ tsp cumin
¼ tsp ground cardamom
1/8 tsp cinnamon
½ tbsp maple syrup
1tbsp olive oil
Kosher salt to taste

Directions

Sauté garlic and onions for 3 minutes on medium heat in the olive oil, add spices and sauté for an additional 3 minutes and add sweet potatoes. Continue cooking for an additional 5 minutes and add almond milk, maple syrup and vegetable stock simmer for 30 minutes till sweet potatoes are tender. Transfer contents to a blender, start on low speed and gradually build to full power to avoid splatter. Blend smooth and season with kosher salt to taste, transfer to container over ice bath to cool properly.

Lentil with Herb Roasted Vegetable Soup
6-8 servings

Ingredients

1/3 lb green lentils
1.5 cup peeled and small diced carrots
1.5 cup small diced white onions
1.5 cup small dice celery
1 cup small diced washed leeks
1 ea bay leaf, dry or fresh
1 tsp chopped oregano
1 tsp chopped chives
1 tsp chopped rosemary
7 cups vegetable stock (see sub recipe)
TT kosher salt
1 tsp ground black pepper
2 tbsp olive oil

Directions

Toss diced vegetables in a bowl with olive oil and chopped herbs. Lay vegetables evenly spread on a baking sheet and roast at 400 degrees for 15 minutes and remove. In a large soup pot combine vegetable stock, bay leaf, pepper and lentils simmer for 20 minutes and add roasted vegetables to the pot, simmer for an additional 20 minutes till lentils are tender, season to taste with kosher salt.

Mushroom with Fresh Thyme Soup
6-8 servings

Ingredients

6 cups Portobello mushrooms, stem removed degilled and diced
4 cups crimini mushrooms, stem removed and diced
1 cup shallots, sliced
2 tbsp garlic, sliced
1 tbsp fresh thyme, picked rough chop
1 cup white wine
6 cups vegetable stock
2 tbsp olive oil
Kosher salt to taste

Directions

Sauté shallots and garlic for three minutes and add mushrooms. Sauté mushrooms till they begin to become tender and add white wine, reduce wine by $3/4^{th}$ and add vegetable stock. Simmer for approximately 25 minutes and transfer contents to blender. Start blender on low to avoid splattering, turn speed to high and season with kosher salt while soup is blending transfer soup to separate container and stir in fresh thyme, cool over ice bath.

Spicy Tofu with Black-Eyed Peas and Braised Chard Soup
6-8 servings

Ingredients
14oz firm tofu, large dice
1.5 cups black-eyed peas, cooked al dente
.5 cup shallots, minced
2 tbsp garlic minced
1 tsp ginger miced
1 bunch green onions, chopped
1 bunch cilantro, chopped
2 tbsp sambal chili sauce
2 tsp sriracha chili sauce
1 tbsp tomato paste
3 cups green Swiss chard chopped
7 cups vegetable stock
2 tbsp fresh lime juice
Kosher salt to taste
1 tbsp olive oil

Directions

Cook black eyed peas in water till they start to turn soft but not too soft, drain water and set aside. In a large soup pot sauté garlic, ginger and shallots in oil for three minutes on medium heat add tomato paste and sauté for another 2 minutes. Pour in the vegetable stock, both chili sauces and black eyed peas. Allow simmering for ten minutes before adding tofu, green onions, cilantro and chard season with fresh lime juice and salt and simmer for 15 more minutes. Salt to taste.

Heirloom Tomato and Smokey Chipotle Soup
6-8 servings

Ingredients

1 tbsp chipotle peppers
4 lbs heirloom tomatoes, chopped
6 ea cloves of garlic
5 ea medium shallots, sliced
2 tbsp olive oil
1 tsp ground cumin
4 cups vegetable stock
Kosher salt to taste

Directions

Sauté shallots and garlic in olive oil for 3 minutes add chipotle and continue to sauté for another 3 minutes. Add tomatoes and simmer till tomatoes start to break down add cumin and vegetable stock simmer for 45 minutes. Transfer to blender and blend till smooth season with salt to taste.

Hot and Spicy Fruit Salad
4-6 servings

Ingredients

1/3 cup orange juice
3 tbsp lime juice
3 tbsp mint, basil or cilantro leaves
$1/4$ tsp red pepper flakes
$1/4$ tsp cayenne pepper
1 tbsp honey or agave nectar
$1/2$ small honeydew melon, cubed
1 papaya or mango, cubed
1 pint strawberries, stems removed and cut in half
1 cup pineapple chunks

Directions

Whisk all ingredients but fruits together and then pour over prepared fruit in large bowl and serve immediately.

This is a great recipe for all of your favorite fruits and you can substitute heat for other spices such as cardamom or cumin.

Desserts and Baked Goods

Ricotta Pumpkin Cheesecake
Serves 8

Ingredients

Filling:
15 oz. container of part skim ricotta
1 cup canned pumpkin (not pumpkin pie mix which is high in sugar)
5 packets of stevia
1 tsp cinnamon
¼ tsp nutmeg
¼ tsp ginger
1/8 tsp cloves
2 tbsp. roasted almonds, crushed into small pieces

Crust:
1 cup ground almond meal flour
2 tablespoons butter
2 tablespoons sugar

Directions

Preheat oven to 350. Melt the butter in the microwave. Combine the sugar and almond flour in a bowl. Pour the butter into the almond mixture and stir until well combined. Place the almond flour dough on the bottom of a nine-inch pie pan. Use your fingers to spread evenly. Bake for 10 minutes, remove from oven to cool.

In a large mixing bowl, combine ricotta, pumpkin, stevia, and pumpkin pie spice and mix well. Spoon filling onto pie crust and top with crushed almonds. Refrigerate for 30 minutes to set.

Basic Spiced Morning Muffin (5 Ways)
Yields 10 muffins

Ingredients

1 cup wheat bran
1 cup whole wheat flour
¼ cup stevia or sugar
1 tsp baking powder
½ tsp baking soda
1 tsp cinnamon
½ tsp nutmeg
½ tsp vanilla extract or almond extract use pure only
Pinch kosher salt
½ cup applesauce (unsweetened) or plain or vanilla yogurt
1 cup almond milk or unsweetened coconut milk
¼ cup vegetable oil
1 egg

Directions

Heat oven to 350 degrees and prepare muffin tin with papers.
In medium bowl combine the dry ingredients and use whisk to mix and distribute evenly.
In large bowl combine wet ingredients.
Add dry ingredients to wet and mix until combined do not overmix.
Using an ice cream scoop or portion scoop, scoop batter into baking cups and bake for 20-22 minutes use a knife or toothpick to check if muffin is done by putting through muffin and pulling out to see if comes out clean if not put in another two minutes and check again until comes out clean.
Let cool about 5 minutes then turn out onto rack for total cool down

Variations

Curry Coconut: add ¾ cup shredded coconut and replace nutmeg with yellow curry and replace the almond milk with coconut milk.

Banana Cardamom: add ½ tsp dry cardamom, ¾ cup mashed overly ripened banana. (option: add ¼ cup mini chocolate chips)

Pumpkin Spice: add 2 tsp pumpkin pie spice instead of cinnamon and nutmeg, substitute applesauce with ½ cup unsweetened canned pumpkin.

Lemon Thyme: replace applesauce with lemon or plain yogurt ½ cup, 1 tbsp dry thyme, ½ pure lemon extract, 1 tsp lemon zest (get this from your lemon using a lemon zester).

*I often reduce wheat bran to ½ cup and adds ½ cup ground almond meal instead or substitute oat bran for wheat bran.

SPICE UP, SLIM DOWN CONTRIBUTOR RECIPES

All of the following recipes have been generously shared by friends, colleagues, and experts, many of whom I have collaborated with over the past decade. The information and formatting varies because in many cases, these recipes are directly from one of their best-selling books so I did not want to modify them in any way. I have included calorie information when available.

Dr. Tanya Altmann, MD

Tanya Altmann, MD, FAAP and Beth Saltz, MPH, RD are best-selling authors of *What to Feed Your Baby*. Dr. Tanya (DrTanya.com) is a UCLA-trained pediatrician, mom of three boys, spokesperson for the American Academy of Pediatrics, health correspondent for local and national news and TV shows and Assistant Clinical Professor at UCLA Mattel Children's Hospital. Beth (nutritioninthekitchen.org) is a registered dietician, chef and mom of two who enjoys developing healthy kid-friendly recipes for her popular blog.

Turmeric Chicken Soup
10-12 servings

Ingredients

2-3 pounds of bone-in, skin-on organic chicken pieces (you can use a whole, cut-up chicken, or just buy drumsticks and thighs, or any combination you prefer)
4 organic carrots, diced
2 stalks organic celery, diced
2 teaspoons kosher salt
1 teaspoon turmeric
1/2 teaspoon white pepper
1 bag fine egg noodles (or brown rice)

Directions

Place chicken pieces in large pot. Add enough water to cover the chicken by about 5 inches. Bring to a boil, then turn the heat down to low. Continue to simmer the soup for 30 minutes.
Carefully remove chicken from the pot. Carefully remove meat from the bones, discarding the skin and keeping the bones aside. You can use two forks to pull the meat off the bones. Or, if you have more time, you can let the chicken cool a little bit and then use gloved hands to pull the meat off. Set chicken aside.
Return the bones to the water and cover pot. Simmer on low another 30-45 minutes.
Remove all bones from pot. Add the carrots, celery, salt, turmeric and white pepper to pot. Stir and simmer 10 minutes.
Meanwhile, cook the egg noodles (or brown rice) in a separate pot, but undercook them by 2 minutes. Drain and set aside.
Start tasting the soup and add more salt and pepper as desired, adding a half-teaspoon of kosher salt as you go. When you like the taste, add the chicken meat back to the broth and heat.
Place noodles into bowls and ladle the soup on top.

Cinnamon Applesauce
6-8 servings

Ingredients

4 golden delicious apples
2 Granny Smith or Envy apples
1 teaspoon cinnamon
¼ cup water
¼ tsp. fresh lemon juice
optional—brown sugar

Directions

Peel and slice the apples, discarding the core. Cut each slice in half. Place cut apples into large microwave-safe bowl. Add the water. Cover with plate and microwave for 5 minutes. Stir and check the apples. Keep cooking, uncovered now, in 2 minute increments. When apples are tender, add the cinnamon and lemon juice to bowl and mix well. Transfer mixture to blender (you can also use a food processor, or even a potato-masher if you like chunky applesauce). Blend just a few seconds, or until you reach the desired texture. Taste. Add ½ to 1 teaspoon brown sugar if desired. Add more lemon juice and cinnamon if desired.

Recipes courtesy of Chef Beth Saltz, MPH, RD, CDE and Tanya Altmann, MD, FAAP authors of What to Feed Your Baby.

Karen Ansel, M.S., R.D.N.

Karen Ansel is a nutrition consultant, spokesperson, journalist and author. She co-wrote and created all the recipes for my third book, The Calendar Diet. Her work has been published in numerous national magazines including *EatingWell, Cooking Light, Prevention, Women's Health, Yoga Journal, Woman's Day* and *O, The Oprah Magazine.* Karen lives with husband, daughters and dogs, Cooper and Cosmo in Long Island, New York. When she's not busy writing about nutrition she loves running, hiking and cooking.

Cardamom Roast Pears with Maple Yogurt
Serves 4

Ingredients

2 Bosc pears, halved and cored
2 teaspoons canola oil
1 large pinch cardamom
1 large pinch sea salt
1 cup nonfat plain Greek yogurt
2 teaspoons maple syrup

Directions

Preheat oven to 400 degrees.
Brush pears with canola oil. Arrange pears on a baking sheet and sprinkle with cardamom and sea salt.
Bake for 25 minutes or until tender. Remove from oven and cool for 10 minutes.
Whisk maple syrup into yogurt.
Arrange pear halves on 4 dessert plates. Top each pear half with a large dollop on yogurt.

Nutrition Stats (per half pear with 2 tablespoons yogurt): 123 calories, 6 g protein, 19 g carbohydrates, 3 g fiber, 13 g sugar, 3 g fat (<1 g sat), 3 mg cholesterol, 82 mg sodium

Jennifer Cohen

Jennifer Cohen is a good friend of mine and a leading fitness authority, best-selling author, entrepreneur and frequent guest on national media. She was recently named in "Greatist" 100 most influential people in Health and Fitness and #16 Most Impactful Fitness Entrepreneurs on Web MD. She has 2 regular columns in Forbes and Entrepreneur and is the lifestyle and fitness spokesperson and consultant for numerous world class. She cofounded of Hot 5, a very popular fitness App and has written two bestselling books, *Strong is the New Skinny* (Random House, 2014) *No Gym Required – Release Your Inner Rock Star* (Key Poter Books, Ltd 2009). She lives in LA with her husband and two young children.

Herbed Salmon
Serves 6-8

Ingredients

2 pounds of skinless salmon filet
1 lemon
Olive oil spray
Salt and pepper to taste
Garlic salt 2 tsp.
Onion salt 2 tsp.
Garlic powder 2 tsp.
Lemon Pepper 2 tsp.
Oregano 2 tsp.
Parsley 2 tsp.
Rosemary 2 tsp.
(feel free to adjust seasoning to your taste preferences)

Directions

Preheat oven to 400 degrees.
Spray broiler pan with olive oil
Place salmon on pan and squeeze lemon on entire filet. Then spray olive oil on top.
Sprinkle sea salt and pepper.
Then sprinkle all the different spices below on filet. Make sure the entire filet is covered well and evenly.
Bake for 35 minutes.

Chef Cat Cora

Cat Cora is a world-renowned chef, author, restaurateur, contributing editor, television host and personality, actress, avid philanthropist, lifestyle entrepreneur and proud mother of six that is best known for her featured role as the first female "Iron Chef" on Food Network's Iron Chef America. She was the first female inducted into The American Academy of Chefs Culinary Hall of Fame. Cat has opened more than 18 restaurants across the U.S. and globally, including: Cat Cora's Kitchen, Ocean by Cat Cora, Cat Cora's Gourmet Market, Kouzzina by Cat Cora at Disney World, CCQ at Macy's, Cat Cora's Taproom, OLILO, Mesa Burger, and her newest addition, Wicked Eats. For more amazing recipes and books, visit her website www.catcora.com or follow her on Instagram: instagram.com/catcora.

Curried Red Snapper with Quinoa and Blanched Chard

This recipe for curried red snapper with quinoa and blanched chard is one of Cat's favorite spice-filled recipes from her book *Cooking from the Hip* (Houghton Mifflin Harcourt, 2007).

Curried Red Snapper
Serves 4-6

Ingredients

2 pounds red snapper fillets
2 teaspoons salt
1 teaspoon black pepper
2 scallions, chopped
3 tablespoons curry powder
2 tablespoons butter
1/4 cup olive oil
1 to 2 Scotch bonnet peppers, seeded and chopped
1 clove garlic, crushed
2 cups coconut milk
1 cup water

2 large tomatoes, roughly chopped
2 medium onions, sliced 1/4-inch thick
10 cilantro sprigs

Directions

Cut the red snapper into small pieces and place in a bowl. Season
with the salt, black pepper, scallion, and curry powder.
Allow the fish to marinate in the refrigerator for at least 1 hour.
When you are ready to proceed, heat the butter and oil in a large
sauté pan. Add the fish and sauté until it is lightly browned on both
sides. Add the peppers, garlic, coconut milk, water, tomatoes, and
onions. Cover the fish and bring to a boil. Reduce the heat, cover the
pan, and simmer until the fish is tender, about 20 to 25 minutes,
adding more water if necessary. Also, add a touch more curry, if
necessary, for your taste. Finish with fresh cilantro leaves and serve
immediately with blanched chard (recipe below) and quinoa cooked
according to package directions.

Blanched Chard
Serves 4

Ingredients

2 lbs Swiss chard
Kosher salt
¼ cup extra-virgin olive oil
2 garlic cloves, thinly sliced
3-4 TBS fresh lemon juice (from 1-2 large lemons)
Freshly ground black pepper

Directions

Fill a large pot with water and place over high heat.
While you're waiting for the water to boil, wash and trim the chard by
cutting away the heavy stems and discarding them. Coarsely chop
the leaves. When the water boils, add 1 TBS salt and the chard.
Cover the pot loosely and cook until the greens are tender, 4-5

minutes.

Carefully pour the greens into a colander and let them drain thoroughly for about 10 minutes.

While the chard is draining, heat a large skillet over medium-high heat and add the olive oil. When the oil is hot but not smoking, add the garlic and cook until lightly browned. Add the chard and sauté until wilted, 2-3 minutes. Add half of the lemon juice and ¼ tsp salt and toss. Taste and add more lemon juice or salt, if you like. Add pepper to taste and serve.

Vivica A. Fox

Vivica A. Fox has achieved a successful career as an actress, producer, entrepreneur and philanthropist. Hollywood screen gem, Fox, has triumphantly built an international brand that stands on the strength that women can do anything. With an extensive body of work that encompasses unforgettable television, stage and film credits, Vivica A. Fox is an inspiration as a Hollywood actress, generous philanthropist and accomplished businesswoman. Even though she appeared as a contestant on Food Network's Worst Cooks in America, battling it out to raise funds for her charity of choice, Best Buddies, Vivica generously let me use one of her favorite recipes for this book.

Vivica's Tasty Tacos
Serves 6-8

Ingredients

1 lb pound of extra lean ground beef or turkey meat
2 white onions , chopped
1 pack taco meat seasoning*
1 pack of pre-shredded cheddar cheese
1 package corn tortillas
2 to 3 large tomatoes, diced
1 large can of sliced black olives

Lettuce, shredded
1-2 cup salsa
½ pint of sour cream
1 can of black beans
1 can of pinto beans.
1-2 tbsp. canola oil + spray
Sea salt and pepper
*Vivica uses Lawry's taco seasoning but there are lots of others out there including lower sodium, organic and gluten-free choices.

Directions

Start by cooking your chopped up onion in canola oil then add your beef or turkey meat. Add Lawry's seasoning salt when meat is browned. Cook your corn tortillas in light canola oil or canola cooking spray to a golden brown crisp add a little bit of cheese to create a crispy shell. Open a can of black beans and pinto beans and cook in a sauce pan add a dash of sea salt and pepper. Chop up your tomatoes, shredded lettuce, black olives and onions and put in serving bowls along wtih your sour cream and salsa. Keep your cooked beef or turkey in a warming dish and corn tortillas on a serving plate covered with a paper towel to absorb excess oil and let your guest create their own tasty tacos.

Chef Elina Fuhrman

Elina Fuhrman is the Author of *Soupelina's Soup Cleanse: Plant-Based Soups + Broths to Heal Your Body, Calm Your Mind, and Transform Your Health* (DaCapo Lifelong , 2016), and Founder + Chef of Soupelina, a mission-driven authentic wellness brand delivering one-of-a-kind plant-based delicious soups + broths that help people eat for their health, heal, prevent and overcome illness. Soupelina's patented recipes are based on the science behind plants, herbs and spices, and their medicinal properties. Formerly, an international journalist for CNN, Elina's fresh approach to healthy eating has made her an inspiring voice on healthy eating and credible wellness expert.

Exotic Spicy Tamarind-Cauliflower Soup
Serves 4-6

> *"I fell in love with tamarind over two decades ago, the moment I took a sip of a refreshing drink that was served to me upon my arrival on the island of Koh Samui, in Thailand. The taste was tangy, delicious and oh so energizing. Years later, I re-discovered tamarind for it's medicinal powers. This pod fruit, popular in South Asia is quite a super food, packed with healing properties and well regarded in Ayurveda. It's excellent for colds, coughs and sore throats."*

Ingredients

4 cups water or Soupelina Lemongrass Cleansing Broth
¼ cup tamarind juice
1 ½ tablespoon red curry paste
1 tablespoon palm sugar
1 ½ tablespoon Tamari
1 package Beech Mushrooms
½ cup daikon rounds
½ cup carrot rounds
1 cup cauliflower, cut into florets
4-5 pods of yardlong bean, cut into 1-inch pieces
½ cup Chinese cabbage, cut
sea salt to taste

Directions

Bring pot of water to boil over medium heat. If using Soupelina Broth, warm the broth until hot over medium-low heat.
Add tamarind juice, sugar, Tamari and salt to achieve a balance of sour, salty and sweet.
Add mushrooms and cook until done for approximately 10-15 minutes.
Add daikon, carrots and cauliflower and cook for another 15-20 minutes until al dente.
Add yardlong bean and cabbage for another 10 minutes.
Remove from heat, let sit for 15-30 minutes for flavors to mature.

Michael Gelman

As Executive Producer of Live with Kelly and Ryan, Michael Gelman is responsible for virtually every aspect of the show. Having taken over the reins of Live in 1987, Michael has the longest tenure at the helm of any of the top syndicated shows. Michael is a father, yogi, skier, tennis addict, wine lover, gardener, techy and lives in New York with his wife, television personality and *Class Mom* author, Laurie Gelman, and their daughters, Jamie and Misha.

Gelman's More is More Guacamole

This guacamole is not just pureed avocado with a couple of tablespoons of flavor. It's almost like an avocado salad. It is overloaded with healthy herbs, vegetables, spices and flavors that people love and that add to the healthfulness of the dish. It even won the grand prize in our beach club competition. The large amount of the tomato also cuts the fat content per serving. You can eat it with regular corn chips, but I prefer either warm soft corn tortillas or bean chips. It's a great accouterment to eggs, sandwiches or anything that needs flavor. I usually make a double recipe so I have leftovers to eat the next few days. It seems to stay green longer because of the larger amount of lime juice in the recipe.

Ingredients

2 avocados – Hass, Medium
1 large red onion
2 large tomatoes
2 Serrano peppers with seeds (or jalapenos) – to taste*
1 medium bunch of cilantro
1-2 limes

Directions

Cut up and mash Avocado.
Tip: Use a fork to make chunkier guacamole!
Chop Tomatoes and finely chop Sweet Red Onions.
Tip: Add more tomatoes for less calories/healthy guacamole!
Finely chop Serrano peppers…Gelman likes his guacamole spicy! He uses the entire pepper, including seeds. (for lower heat, omit seeds)

Tip: Use gloves to protect your hands, which end up touching your eyes and other sensitive body parts.

Tip: Misconception that only seeds are hot…ribs and veins are hotter. White parts = hot!

Tip: Scoville Heat Units (SHU): Jalapeño 2,500-8,000...Serrano 10,000-23,000. You can use jalapeño as substitute.

Roughly chop Cilantro, some stems are OK.

Lime and Salt…squeeze fresh lime juice and use very coarse sea salt to taste.

*If you don't want to use Serrano peppers, Michael suggests using Tabasco-style hot sauce to taste instead.

Dr. Suzanne Gilberg-Lenz, MD

Dr. Gilberg-Lenz almost delivered my first son, Max. She was on call when I went in for an emergency C-section. We got to know each other during my hospitalization and have been good friends ever since. She is a board certified ob-gyn and integrative doctor who loves herbal medicine, meditation, chilling at the Korean spa with her girls, yoga, exploring historic Los Angeles neighborhood's, the art of storytelling and cooking with her 2 kids, when they aren't rolling their eyes so hard at her that they can hardly stand.

Kitchari
Serves 4

This is a classic Ayurvedic comfort & healing food - a wonderful complete protein with lots of spices that aid in digestion. This recipe was generously shared by Suzanne's friend and Ayurvedic Practitioner Anjali Deva.

Ingredients

1 tsp black mustard seeds
1 tsp cumin seeds
1 small pinch asafoetida (also known as Hing) powder (optional)
2 tsp turmeric powder
2 tsp cumin powder

2 tsp coriander powder
2 tablespoons ghee or oil of choice
1 cup split yellow mung dal, rinsed well, soaked overnight, and drained
1 cup white basmati rice, rinsed well and drained
1/2 inch piece of ginger, diced
1 leek, diced - can be replaced with onion or shallot

Directions

In a soup pot, combine dal and rice. Add water to 1 inch above the lentil and grain level.
Bring to a boil. Once at a rolling boil, add in the turmeric, coriander, cumin and Hing powders and stir in evenly. Reduce heat to simmer, stirring occasionally.
In a separate pan, heat the ghee or oil over medium heat. Add in mustard seeds, when they begin to pop add in the cumin seeds, ginger and leek. Sauté over medium heat until the leeks are translucent (about 10-15 minutes).
Add the sauté to the rice and lentil mixture. Continue to cook until the lentils and rice are evenly cooked, this can take anywhere from 30-50 minutes. You may have to experiment with the amount of water you use to find the right consistency for you (the more water, the thinner the consistency). If you find the water is running low and the grains are sticking to the bottom of the pan, add in more hot water.
*You may also choose to add some of your favorite vegetables half way.

Mireille Guiliano

Mireille Guiliano is the author of *French Women Don't Get Fat: The Secret of Eating for Pleasure*, the #1 *New York Times* bestseller. I had the pleasure of meeting Mireille over a decade ago while filming Fit TV's Diet Doctor and we have been friends ever since. A former chief executive at LVMH (Clicquot Inc.), she has been called "the high priestess of French lady wisdom" (*USA Today*), " an ambassador of France and its art of living" (*Le Figaro*), "an idea entrepreneur"

(*Harvard Business Review*) and "an art-of-living guru" (*The New York Times*). Guiliano is also the author of *French Women for All Seasons; Women, Work & The Art of Savoir Faire; The French Women Don't Get Fat Cookbook; French Women Don't Get Facelifts* and *Meet Paris Oyster*. Born in France, she "ages with style and attitude" in New York City, Paris and Provence. For additional information and a more detailed biography go to mireilleguiliano.com

Curried Chicken with Cucumber
Serves 4

Ingredients

1 tablespoon unsalted butter
1 tablespoon olive oil
4 (6-to-8 ounce) skinless, boneless chicken breasts, cut lengthwise into ½ inch strips
Salt and freshly ground pepper
½ cup crème fraiche
1 tablespoon curry powder
2 seedless cucumbers, washed and cut into ½ inch slices
Juice of 1 lemon
Cooked basmati rice for serving

Directions

Heat the butter and olive oil in a large skillet over medium-high heat. Season the chicken with salt and pepper and add to the skillet. Cook until golden, stirring occasionally, about 10 minutes.
Meanwhile, in a medium bowl, combine the crème fraiche, curry, and cucumber slices and set aside.
When the chicken is golden, deglaze the pan with lemon juice, scraping up all the brown bits from the bottom of the pan. Add the cucumber mixture and stir to combine. Cook for about 3 minutes or until the cucumbers are al dente. Season to taste and serve with basmati rice.

Lentils Three Ways: Soup, Side, & Salad
Serves 4

Ingredients

1 teaspoon extra-virgin olive oil, plus additional for serving
2 garlic cloves, peeled and minced
1 shallot, peeled and minced
1 teaspoon fresh thyme (or rosemary)
10 ounces lentils (preferably the tiny green variety, Puy), washed and picked over
1 tablespoon curry powder
3¾ cups water
2 cups hot vegetable stock (if making as a soup)
Coarse salt and freshly ground pepper
Crème fraiche for garnishing soup (optional)

Directions

Warm the olive oil in a heavy saucepan over medium heat. Add the garlic, shallot, and thyme, and sauté, stirring, until fragrant and softened, about 2 minutes.
Add the lentils, curry powder, and freshly ground pepper and cook, stirring, for 1 minute.
Add the water, increase heat to medium-high, and bring mixture to a boil. Lower heat, cover with lid, and simmer for 35 to 40 minutes.
To serve the lentils as a soup, add hot vegetable stock during the last 10 minutes of cooking. When lentils are tender, carefully transfer half of the mixture to a blender or food mill and puree until smooth and creamy. Return the pureed soup to the saucepan and stir to combine. This creates a creamy lentil soup with some texture. Season to taste and serve hot, garnished with a dollop of crème fraiche and a sprinkle of curry powder, if desired. To serve the lentils as a side dish, drain any remaining water once the lentils are tender and place in a serving bowl. Season with coarse salt to taste and a drizzle of olive oil and serve immediately. You can add your favorite chopped fresh herbs as well.
Note: Any leftovers will make for a delicious salad over the next 2-3 days. Simply take the lentils out of the refrigerator 15 minutes before

using and create a salad of your choice with some lettuce leaves, the lentils, and any other raw veggies you wish to add. If you would like to serve the salad as a main course or complete meal, 1 or 2 soft-boiled eggs are a lovely addition, as is a small can of tuna or sardines or some leftover cooked salmon.

Dr. Sanjay Gupta

Dr. Sanjay Gupta is a practicing neurosurgeon and CNN's Chief Medical Correspondent. He is the author of three best-selling books: *Chasing Life*, *Cheating Death* and *Monday Mornings*. Gupta is married with three daughters, for whom he always cooks Sunday morning breakfast and Turmeric Tea.

Dr. Sanjay Gupta's Calming Turmeric Tea
1 serving

Ingredients

1 cup almond milk
½ tsp. turmeric
1 tsp. cinnamon
¼ tsp. ginger
1 tsp. honey

Directions

Heat almond milk in microwave.
Stir in turmeric, cinnamon and ginger.
Drizzle honey on top and enjoy!

66 calories

Chef Johnny Iuzzini

Johnny Iuzzini is a pastry Chef, author, and TV personality. A graduate of the Culinary Institute of America in Hyde Park, he has worked at world class restaurants including Daniel, Café Boulud, and Jean Georges, where he became Executive Pastry Chef at just 26 years old. In May 2002, he was named "Best New Pastry Chef" by New York and in May 2006, the James Beard Foundation awarded Johnny "Outstanding Pastry Chef of the Year. Johnny's first cookbook, *Dessert Four Play: Sweet Quartets From a Four-Star Pastry Chef*, was published in 2008 and his second book *Sugar Rush: Master Tips, Techniques, and Recipes for Sweet Baking* was published in 2014. Johnny was the head judge of Bravo's culinary competition series "Top Chef Just Desserts" for two seasons. He was co-judge with Mary Berry in ABC's "The Great Holiday Baking Show." Since leaving Restaurant Jean Georges, Johnny has started his own pastry consulting company, aptly named Sugar Fueled Inc. and is a Chef Ambassador for Family Reach Foundation. In May of 2017, Johnny realized his dream of making his own chocolate by launching *Chocolate by Johnny Iuzzini*, delicious hand-made, single origin, bean-to-bar chocolates. I did an event with Johnny several years ago and we had a blast cooking healthful dessert recipes together (to be clear, he cooked and I talked about the healthful properties of what he was cooking!)

Macerated Strawberries *(from Sugar Rush)*
Makes About 1 ½ Cups

Directions

Hull and quarter about 12 ripe strawberries. Drizzle about 1 teaspoon (20g) honey and 1 teaspoon (5 g) balsamic vinegar over them. Add a little chopped fresh tarragon and finely grated lemon zest. Toss well and let stand for about 10 minutes. Before using, squeeze a few drops of fresh lemon juice over the berries and toss.

Stewed Blueberries *(from Sugar Rush)*
Makes About 1 Cup

Directions

Heat about 1/3 cup (80 g) orange juice in a small saucepan with a pinch of sugar and a small piece of cinnamon stick until warm. Add 1 cup (140 g) blueberries and heat for 3 to 4 minutes, stirring frequently, until the liquid begins to pop. Do not overcook then or they will release pectin and get gummy. Stir in some finely grated orange zest and use warm or at room temperature.

Spiced Walnuts (from *Dessert Four Play*)
Makes About 1 1/3 Cups

Ingredients

For the Spice Mix:
3 Cinnamon Sticks, Broken Into Pieces
6 Allspice Berries
1 ¼ Teaspoons (5 g) Black Peppercorns
4 Whole Cloves
17 Cardamom Seeds
2 Star Anise
1/8 Teaspoon (0.4 g) Ground Mace
1/8 Teaspoon (0.5 g) Coarse Salt

For the Walnuts:
3 Tablespoons (42 g) Unsalted Butter
4 Ounces (113 g) Walnut Halves
1 Tablespoon (6 g) Spice Mix

Directions

Combine all the spices with the salt in a spice grinder and grind to a fine powder. Sift, then store for up to 3 months in a glass jar out of the light.
Melt the butter in a skillet over medium heat. When the butter foams,

add the nuts and cook, stirring often, until the nuts are fragrant and toasted, about 3 minutes.

Scrape into a strainer so all the excess butter can drip off. Transfer to a bowl and toss the nuts with the spice mix.

Let cool completely and store in an airtight container for up to 3 days.

Dr. Timothy S. Harlan, MD, FACP

Dr. Harlan is a practicing, board-certified Internist. He is the Executive Director of the Goldring Center for Culinary Medicine, the first working teaching kitchen at a medical school, and is the force behind Dr. Gourmet (www.DrGourmet.com), a leading evidence-based health information and healthy recipe website.

Peruvian Chicken
6 servings

Ingredients

2 jalapeno peppers
1 cup cilantro
4 cloves garlic (divided)
2 Tbsp. reduced fat mayonnaise
1/4 cup reduced fat sour cream
2 Tbsp. olive oil (divided)
1/2 lime (juiced)
1 tsp. lime zest
1/4 tsp. salt
to taste fresh ground black pepper
1 Tbsp. ground cumin
1 Tbsp. paprika
1/2 tsp. fresh ground black pepper
1/2 tsp. dried oregano
4 tsp. reduced sodium soy or tamari sauce
1 whole chicken (about 1 1/2 pounds)

Directions

To make the sauce, place the peppers, cilantro, 2 cloves of garlic, mayonnaise, sour cream, 1 tablespoon olive oil, lime juice, lime zest, salt, and fresh ground black pepper to taste in a blender and puree until smooth.
Place in the refrigerator to chill.
Preheat the oven to 325°F.
Mince the remaining 2 cloves of garlic and place in a large mixing bowl.
Add the cumin, paprika, 1/2 teaspoon black pepper, oregano, 1 tablespoon olive oil, and the soy sauce to the bowl.
Blend well.
Split the chicken in half and coat thoroughly with the rub.
Place both halves of the chicken on a roasting rack, skin side up, and roast for about 60 minutes until the internal temperature is 160°F at the center of the breast.
Remove from the oven and let rest for about 5 minutes. Cut into 8 pieces – two wings, two thighs and four breast pieces.
Serve topped with the green sauce.

*This recipe can easily be multiplied and makes very good leftovers.

Calories 311, Total Fat 20g, Saturated Fat 5g, Monounsaturated Fat 7g, Cholesterol 106mg, Sodium 284mg, Total Carbohydrates 2g, Dietary Fiber 0g, Sugars 1g, Protein 28g

Kimberly Jung

Kimberly is the CEO & Co-founder, Rumi Spice, a company started by former Army officers who served combat tours in Afghanistan. Since leaving the military, the cofounders felt they still had unfinished business to support Afghanistan and its people. They founded Rumi Spice to work directly with Afghan farmers to import exceptionally high quality saffron. In Afghanistan, they've hired 384 Afghan women, stood up our three processing facilities, and have over 90 farmers in their network. They make up 3.6% of Afghanistan's total foreign direct investment in agriculture. Rumi saffron now graces the tables and kitchens of The French Laundry, Daniel, Le Bernardin, Bouley, and the Culinary Institute of America and retails stores include Dean & Deluca, Whole Foods, and Central Markets. Rumi aired on Shark Tank May 5 and received an offer from Mark Cuban. To learn more about Rumi Spice visit their website rumispice.com.

Saffron Herb Pistachio Rice
Yields 4 cups of rice

Ingredients

2 cups rice
2 1/3 cups boiling water
1 tsp saffron threads soaked in 3 tbsp water OR 3-4 tbsp Rumi saffron butter
1/2 cup chopped raisins soaked in lemon juice for half an hour
1 oz fresh dill
1/2 oz fresh tarragon
1/2 cup toasted coarsely chopped pistachios

Directions

Melt the butter, coat the rice, then add the boiling water, salt and pepper (and saffron) and steam with lid tightly on low heat for 12 to 15 minutes.
Cool and break apart rice grains. Chop all the herbs and add just before serving with the raisins.
Mix well then sprinkle pistachios on top. Enjoy!

Dean Karnazas

Ultra marathoner and NY Times bestselling author, Dean Karnazes was named by TIME magazine as one of the "100 Most Influential People in the World." He lives with his family in the San Francisco. I have known Dean for over a decade and I was thrilled when he agreed to contribute and was so passionate about spices. Here is what he shared with me:

"Being Greek, I love to entertain. I always make morning coffee for the household and for our guests. I'm usually up earliest so it makes sense. One unusual thing I do is to grind sprigs of wild rosemary with the coffee. I pick some from our garden and it has an incredible mellowing effect on the coffee's flavor, yet with quite powerful results. Rosemary has one of the highest ORAC values of anything on earth! Fresh rosemary is ideal, but even dried rosemary seems to neutralize coffees' acidity and leave you feeling especially alert and energized. On the theme of my Greek heritage, one lesser-known spice that I incorporate into many dishes is ground fenugreek. The taste is rich and flavorful, and fenugreek works wonders for speeding post-marathon recovery. Here is one of my favorite recipes."

Ikarian Cauliflower with Ginger & Fenugreek
Serves 4 - 6

Ingredients

2 tablespoons olive oil
1 teaspoon mustard seeds
1 medium sized red onion, diced
1 teaspoons freshly grated ginger
1 medium sized cauliflower chopped
1/2 teaspoon turmeric
1/2 teaspoon red chili powder
Sea salt to taste
2 tomatoes, chopped
1 tablespoon dried fenugreek
2 tablespoons unflavored yogurt (or vegan yogurt)
1 packet stevia
Cilantro to finish

Directions

Heat the oil on medium heat for about 1 minute.
Add the mustard seeds and heat until the seeds begin to crackle.

Add in the onion and the ginger and sauté for 3 to 4 minutes.
Add in the cauliflower and cover and cook for 3 minutes.
Mix in the turmeric, chili powder and salt and stir well.
Add in the tomatoes and cover and cook for five minutes.
Remove the cover and stir well.
Mix in the dried fenugreek, yogurt and the stevia and cover and cook
for another five minutes until the vegetables are nice and soft.
Stir in the cilantro and serve.

Ashley Koff, RD

Ashley Koff is your better health enabler. To help patients get and
keep better health results, Ashley developed better nutrition tools to
assess their current nutrition and determine what their bodies need to
run better. Today those tools are available online as part of *The Better
Nutrition Membership*. A practitioner first, Ashley is an award-winning
nutrition expert, author, speaker, consultant, spokesperson and
advocate. She regularly shares her better nutrition message with
millions via national media, social media and co-hosts the podcast
"Take Out with Ashley and Robyn." For more about Ashley or to get
the Better Nutrition tools visit AshleyKoffApproved.com.

Better Hemp Pesto
Serves 6-8

Ashley shares "While I love pesto, I love hemp pesto even more and
you will too! This pesto packs plant protein and essential fatty acids,
fiber, iron, magnesium, manganese and more. This doesn't pack
carbs, so pair it with your favorite carb or enjoy it with non-starchy
veggies as part of a lower carb pit stop."

Ingredients

2 cups fresh basil leaves, tightly packed
2 tablespoons hemp seeds
2 tablespoons cashews, soaked

1 small garlic clove, roughly chopped
½ teaspoon lemon zest
¼ teaspoon sea salt
1 teaspoon lemon juice
3 tablespoons extra virgin olive oil

Directions

In a food processor, combine basil, hemp, cashews, garlic, lemon zest and juice. Pulse to roughly combine. With motor running, slowly pour in 3 tablespoons of olive oil. Process until mixture is smooth, about 10-15 seconds. You will likely need to stop and wipe the edges of the blender or food processor and then resume pureeing.

Better Turmeric Pear Toast

From Ashley: "Heard turmeric is a better choice? It is because it helps promote a healthy inflammatory response which makes it great for hard workout recovery, great for better skin as well as to keep colds and illness away. Enjoy it here to complement the flavor and health benefits of pear. This one is nutrient-balanced so it's a stand-alone pit stop or a great appetizer at brunch. I love cacao. It is not only delicious, but also rich in magnesium! Magnesium is nature's anti-stress mineral. It will help you relax better, digest better, and therefore absorb nutrients better. Check out my Better Magnesium Menu for more magnesium-rich recipe ideas."

Ingredients

3 tsp Gaia Herbs Golden Milk powder
1 Tbsp raw cacao nibs
1 pear, sliced
2 Tbsp cashew butter

Directions

Using two teaspoons, spoon cashew butter onto pear slices. Sprinkle golden milk powder. Top with cacao nibs and enjoy!

Chef John La Puma, MD

Dr. John La Puma MD, a board-certified internist and professionally trained chef in Santa Barbara, California, is the founder of ChefMD and Chef Clinic. With Michael Roizen MD of the Cleveland Clinic, he taught the first culinary medicine course in a U.S. medical school, in 2003. Dr. La Puma currently runs an urban organic educational farm studying nature and food as medicine. This salmon recipe is from his *ChefMD's Big Book of Culinary Medicine* (Harmony, 2008) and the baked apple is from Dr. La Puma and Roizen's *Cooking the RealAge Way* (HarperCollins, 2003).

Cumin-Crusted Salmon Over Silky Sweet Potatoes
4 servings

Ingredients

2 large or 3 medium sweet potatoes, scrubbed and cut into 3/4-inch chunks (about 1 ½ pounds)
2 teaspoons cumin seeds
2 teaspoons ground cardamom
¾ teaspoon salt
4 5-ounce fresh Alaskan king salmon fillets, skin on
½ cup packaged sweet potato soup
2 tablespoons pepitas (pumpkin seeds), toasted

Directions

Preheat the oven to 425° F. Steam or microwave the sweet potatoes in a medium bowl until very tender (8 to 10 minutes for steamed, 4 to 5 minutes for microwaved).
Sprinkle the cumin seeds, cardamom, and ¼ teaspoon of the salt over the meaty sides of the salmon. Heat a large oven-proof non-stick skillet over medium-high heat until hot. Coat with cooking spray.
Add the salmon, seasoned sides down; cook for 3 minutes or until browned. Turn the fillets over; place the skillet in the oven, and bake for 8 to 10 minutes or until the salmon is opaque in the center.
Add the soup and the remaining ½ teaspoon salt to the hot cooked

sweet potatoes. Mash with a potato masher to desired consistency. Transfer to serving plates; top with the salmon and pepitas.

Substitutions: Butternut squash soup may replace the sweet potato soup, and toasted sliced almonds may replace the pepitas.

Tip: For a spicier flavor, add 1 teaspoon chipotle hot pepper sauce, such as Tabasco brand, or ¼ teaspoon cayenne pepper to the sweet potatoes.

406 calories per serving, Total Fat: 15.9 g, Saturated Fat: 2.6 g, Fiber: 5.8 g, Carbohydrates: 39.9 g, Sugar: 7.4 g, Protein: 27.2 g, Sodium: 636.7 mg

Sweet Baked Apples with Cherries and Citrus
Serves 4

A great natural source of vitamin C, citrus fruits add freshness, sprightliness, and flavor, making your real age 1.1 days younger.

Ingredients

2 large baking apples, such as Rome Beauty
1¼ cups apple juice, preferably organic unfiltered, divided ½ cup (2 ounces) dried pitted cherries
¼ teaspoon ground cloves
2 seedless clementines or tangerines, peeled, separated into segments
Mint sprigs (optional)

Directions

Heat oven to 400 degrees. Cut apples in half; cut out and discard core, seeds, and stems. Place ¼ cup of the apple juice in an 8-inch baking dish or casserole. Place apples cut side down over juice. Bake 15 to 18 minutes or until apples are tender. Meanwhile, simmer remaining 1 cup apple juice in a small saucepan over medium-high heat 5 minutes. Add cherries and cloves; reduce heat and simmer uncovered 10 minutes, or until cherries are plumped, stirring occasionally. Remove from heat; stir in citrus sections. Arrange apple halves cut sides up on serving dishes. Pour any remaining liquid from dish into cherry mixture and spoon the mixture over apples. Garnish with mint sprigs, if desired.

Tips: A little ground clove goes a long way—its zippiness is a perfect complement to this fall/winter dessert. Try studding each apple with 2 whole cloves, so that they are submerged in the apple juice as the apples bake. Remove the clove before eating the apple, which will now be scented with zingy spice. This is an early summer treat as that is when cherries are at their best.

Substitutions: Dried cranberries may replace the cherries. Baking apples cook more quickly and develop a softer texture when baked than eating apples. McIntosh apples are another good choice.

Dr. Zhaoping Li MD, PhD

Dr. Li is the Director of the Center for Human Nutrition, Chief of the Division of Clinical Nutrition and Lynda and Stewart Resnick Endowed Chair in Human Nutrition at David Geffen School of Medicine at the UCLA. She is not only a colleague but also a good friend and I respect her tremendously. Dr. Li is currently vice-President of National Board of Physician Nutrition Specialist, President of the World Association of Chinese Doctors in Clinical Nutrition, and a member of ASN Medical Nutrition Council. Dr. Li is board certified in Internal Medicine and as a Physician Nutrition Specialist. She has been Principal Investigator for over 50 investigator-initiated NIH and industry- sponsored clinical trials and published over 150 peer-reviewed papers.

Lemon-Barley Pilaf with Chicken and Thyme
Serves 4

Fluffy barley is combined with chicken, lemon and thyme flavors for a delicious, comforting healthy meal.

Ingredients

4 tablespoons olive oil, divided
1 large shallot, minced
1 medium garlic, minced
3/4 cup pearl barley
2-1/4 cups chicken broth
1 bay leaf
2 celery ribs, cut into 1/2-inch dice
1 medium carrot, peeled, cut into 1/2-inch dice
1 teaspoon grated lemon zest
3 tablespoon lemon juice, divided
Kosher salt and freshly ground black pepper
4 (5 ounce) chicken breasts, skinless and boneless
1/2 cup dry white wine
1/4 cup chicken broth, low-sodium
2 tablespoon minced thyme leaves

Directions

Preheat an oven to 400 degrees and position an oven rack in the center. Place a medium heavy saucepan on the stove over a moderate heat. Add 2 tablespoons of oil and when shimmering, add the shallot and cook until tender, about 3 minutes. Add the garlic and cook until fragrant, about 1 minute. Add the barley and cook, stirring constantly, until well coated in the shallot and garlic, about 2 minutes. Add 2 cups of chicken broth and bay leaf and bring the liquid to a boil. Reduce the heat to low, stir and cover. Cook until the barley is almost tender with a slight bite, about 25 minutes. Stir in the celery and carrot and cook until the vegetables are tender, about 5 minutes. Remove the barley pilaf from the heat, stir and remove bay leaf. Add the lemon zest and 1 tablespoon of juice, taste and season with salt and pepper. While the barley is cooking, place a large nonstick skillet on the stove and add the remaining oil. Season the chicken with salt and pepper. When the oil is shimmering, carefully add the chicken, top side first, until golden-brown, about 3 minutes. Using tongs, flip chicken breast and transfer to the oven to bake until cooked through and registers 165 degrees on an instant-read thermometer, about 8 to 10 minutes. When cooked, transfer chicken to a cutting board, cover loosely with foil and rest until ready to carve.

Place the skillet on top the stove over a moderate-high heat. Add the white wine and cook until almost dry, about 4 minutes. Add the broth and thyme leaves and cook until thickened, about 2 minutes. Remove from heat, taste and season with salt and pepper.

To serve: Divide the pilaf between 4 warmed plates. Carve chicken, arrange over the barley, spoon sauce over chicken and serve immediately.

Oven-Roasted Cod with Tomato Jam, Feta and Olives
Serves 4

This Greek-inspired dish is a simple and easy dinner solution for a busy weeknight but works well for entertaining too. Any firm-fleshed white fish will work here, including halibut, cod, or mahi-mahi. Make an extra batch of the tomato jam, which is terrific spread on bread or used as a dip.

Ingredients

1-1/2 pounds ripe plum tomatoes, cored and coarsely chopped
1/4 cup honey
3 tablespoons plus 1/4 cup freshly squeezed lemon juice, divided
2 tablespoons tomato paste
2 tablespoons cider vinegar
1 tablespoon finely minced garlic
2 teaspoons kosher salt, plus more as needed
1 teaspoon dried oregano
1/2 teaspoon dried cumin
1/2 teaspoon freshly ground black pepper
1/4 teaspoon dried red pepper flakes
1/4 cup extra-virgin olive oil, plus more for coating pan
3 cloves garlic, peeled and sliced thin
1/3 cup dry white wine
1/4 cup freshly squeezed lemon juice
2 tablespoons chopped fresh thyme leaves, plus more for garnish
1-1/2 cups mixed green and black brine-cured olives, pitted
4 (5 to 6 ounce) cod fillets, or other firm white fish
Freshly ground white pepper

1/3 cup crumbled feta cheese, for serving

Directions

To prepare tomato jam, place tomatoes, honey, 3 tablespoons lemon juice, tomato paste, cider vinegar, garlic, salt, oregano, cumin, black pepper, and red pepper flakes in a large saucepan. Heat over medium-high heat until mixture boils. Reduce heat to medium-low and simmer, stirring occasionally, until mixture reduces and thickens to a jam-like consistency, about 60 to 75 minutes. Remove from heat and cool completely.

Preheat oven to 425 degrees and place a rack in the center. In a large saucepan, place olive oil and heat over medium heat. Add garlic and cook, stirring frequently, until light golden, about 3 to 4 minutes. Add wine, remaining 1/4 cup lemon juice, and 1/2 cup tomato jam and stir well. Simmer tomato mixture until slightly reduced and thickened, about 6 to 8 minutes. Remove pan from heat and stir in thyme leaves and olives.

Coat the bottom of a ceramic baking dish large enough to hold the fish with a thin film of olive oil. Season fillets on both sides with salt and pepper. Place fish in the prepared pan and cover with tomato mixture. Cover baking dish and place in preheated oven. Roast until fish just begins to flake, about 12 to 15 minutes.

To serve, transfer fish using a fish spatula to individual shallow serving bowls. Spoon about 4 to 6 ounces of tomato mixture on and around fish. Top with tomato jam and sprinkle with feta cheese. Serve immediately.

Lisa Lillien

My good pal Lisa Lillien (a.k.a. Hungry Girl) is a *New York Times* best-selling author and the creator of the Hungry Girl brand. She is the founder of hungry-girl.com, the free daily email service that entertains and informs hungry people everywhere. Lisa is the author of twelve bestselling cookbooks, six of which debuted at #1 on the *New York Times* Best Sellers list. She has also starred in a top-rated cooking show on both Food Network and Cooking Channel. A self-proclaimed "mad scientist" in the kitchen, Lisa dishes out guilt-free recipes, tips & tricks, supermarket finds, and survival guides for real-world eating situations.

Slow-Cooker Chicken Burrito Bonanza
Serves 4

Ingredients

1 ½ lbs. raw boneless skinless chicken breast
¼ tsp. black pepper
½ tsp. salt
1 cup chopped onion
One 15-oz. can black beans, drained and rinsed
One 14.5-oz. can diced tomatoes, drained
One 4-oz. can diced green chiles, drained
1 ½ cups reduced-sodium chicken broth
1 tbsp. chili powder
1 tbsp. ground cumin
½ tsp. onion powder
½ tsp. garlic powder
½ tsp. paprika
4 cups cauliflower rice/crumbles
½ cup shredded reduced-fat Mexican-blend cheese
Optional seasonings: additional salt and black pepper

Directions

Place chicken in a slow cooker, and season with pepper and ¼ tsp. salt. Top with onion, beans, tomatoes, and chiles.
Add broth and seasonings, including remaining ¼ tsp. salt. Gently stir.
Cover and cook on high for 3 – 4 hours or on low for 7 – 8 hours, until chicken is fully cooked.
Transfer chicken to a large bowl. Shred with two forks.

Return shredded chicken to the slow cooker, and mix well.

Add cauliflower rice/crumbles, and stir to mix.

If cooking on low heat, increase heat to high. Cover and cook for 55 minutes, or until cauliflower is tender.

Serve with a slotted spoon, draining the liquid. Top each serving with 1 tbsp. cheese.

214 calories, 4.5 g total fat (1.5 g sat fat), 640 mg sodium, 18 g carbs, 5.5 g fiber, 4.5 g sugars, 26 g protein

Tracey Mallett

Tracey is an acclaimed International Fitness and Wellness Expert, dancer, choreographer and Master Pilates Instructor. Mallett owns her own fitness and Pilates studio in Los Angeles, and is currently certifying trainers worldwide in her program bootybarre and bbarreless. Her workouts have appeared in dozens of publications including Prevention, Shape, Fitness Magazine, Women's Health, the Los Angeles Times, Pilates Style and Self and she appears regularly on TV including Good Morning New York, The Style Network for E! Entertainment, Access Hollywood, KTLA's Morning Show, KABC and others. She also appeared on Ellen joining First Lady Michelle Obama, Ellen DeGeneres, and a group of excited school children in an exercise routine developed by Mallett as part of the "Let's Move" campaign. Born in the United Kingdom, and now resides in Pasadena, California with her husband and their two amazing children Amber and Ty. We met a few years ago through a mutual friend and have had a blast working on a few projects together. These recipes are from bootybarreBURN.com

Broccoli Cheese Frittata
Serves 1

Serving suggestion: Serve with a green salad dressed with olive oil and seasoned rice vinegar dressing, or serve with Asian Cole Slaw.

Ingredients

Nonfat olive oil spray
2 tablespoons chopped onions
1 clove garlic, chopped
¼ cup chopped red bell pepper
½ cup chopped broccoli
½ cup chopped Roma tomato
¼ teaspoon fresh basil, chopped
1 whole egg
3 egg whites
Salt and pepper, to taste
Pinch red pepper flakes
½ cup shredded part-skim mozzarella or reduced fat Monterey Jack cheese

Preheat the oven to 350 degrees. Heat an 8-inch nonstick pan with the olive oil spray. Sauté onions, garlic, bell pepper, and broccoli over low heat until the onions are translucent and the vegetables are tender. Add tomatoes and basil and stir. Beat the eggs together with the salt and pepper and pour over the vegetables. Stir briefly and cook just until sides are set, about two to three minutes, or until the frittata gets puffy an the eggs are set but still moist.

Turkey Burger with Ranch Dressing
Serves 4

Serving suggestion: Serve each portion with an apple cut into wedges and sprinkled with cinnamon.

Ingredients

1 pound (16 ounces) fresh ground turkey meat
2 egg whites, lightly beaten
¼ cup whole-grain breadcrumbs (such as Ezekiel bread)
1 tablespoon Dijon mustard
1 teaspoon dried thyme
1 teaspoon dried oregano
½ teaspoon garlic powder
1/8 teaspoon cayenne pepper
¼ teaspoon salt

Directions

In a medium-sized bowl, mix together all the ingredients. Divide the mixture into four equal parts and form each portion into a patty. These patties may be cooked immediately or frozen to use later.
1 4-ounce turkey burger
1 slice reduced-fat cheese
2 slices or ½ cup of tomato
1 romaine lettuce leaf
1 whole-wheat bun

Dressing

1 teaspoon reduced-fat mayonnaise
1 teaspoon low-fat Greek yogurt
1/8 teaspoon garlic powder

Kristin McGee

Kristin McGee is a celebrity yoga and Pilates teacher author of CHAIR YOGA and a mom to 9 month old twins and a toddler. Instead of just giving me a recipe, Kristin share her 'day of spices' with me.

Wake up and have breakfast usually eggs which I scramble with some fresh spinach and top with cayenne and turmeric cracker pepper and some fresh avocado.

Mid-morning snack Greek yogurt with blueberries and some walnuts sprinkled with cinnamon.

Lunch is Open faced turkey sprinkled with curry powder and a side of black bean soup sprinkled with cumin.

Dinner is Greek chicken marinade.

Greek Chicken Marinade
Serves 2

1/2 teaspoon Juice of one lemon
Tablespoon dried Oregano
Tablespoon Fresh chopped dill
Teaspoon salt
Teaspoon pepper
2 organic chicken breasts
Marinate in a ziploc bag in fridge all day.
Grill or bake
Serve with black olives, hummus, tzatziki, tomatoes, lettuce and cucumber (pita bread option).

Natalie Morales

Natalie Morales, wife and mother of two boys, is the West Coast anchor of NBC's *TODAY* show, host of *Access Hollywood*, and cohost of *Access Hollywood Live*. She previously served as news anchor and cohost of *TODAY*'s third hour. She lives in Los Angeles, California. This recipe is from her upcoming book, *At Home with Natalie* (Houghton Mifflin Harcourt, April 2018)

Moroccan Turkey Chili
Serves 8 to 10
Gluten – Free

2 tablespoons extra-virgin olive oil
1 medium yellow onion, diced
2 cloves garlic, minced
2 pounds lean ground turkey
Kosher salt and freshly ground black pepper
2 tablespoons Ras El Hanout (spice blend)
2 tablespoons chili powder
1 teaspoon ground cinnamon
1 teaspoon ground cumin
1 teaspoon dried oregano
2 sweet potatoes, peeled and cut into ½-inch pieces
1 (28-ounce) can diced tomatoes with juices
2 cups chicken broth
1 cup water
2 tablespoons tomato paste
½ red bell pepper, cut into ½-inch chunks
½ yellow bell pepper, cut into ½-inch chunks
2 stalks celery, cut into ½-inch pieces
1 zucchini, cut into 1-inch cubes
1 (12-ounce) can cannellini beans, drained and rinsed
1 (12-ounce) can chickpeas, drained and rinsed
Pinch red pepper flakes (optional)
½ cup chopped fresh cilantro, for garnish

In a slow cooker or large skillet (if you're using a slow cooker set first to sauté function, and if you don't have a sauté option, then use a skillet), warm the olive oil over medium-high heat. Add the onion and garlic and cook, stirring, until the onion is translucent, 5 to 7 minutes. Add the ground turkey and cook, stirring, until lightly browned, 6 to 8 minutes. Season with salt and pepper to taste. Turn the slow cooker to high (transfer everything to the slow cooker now, if you've been using a skillet), add the Ras el Hanout, chili powder, cinnamon, cumin, and oregano and stir into the meat letting it all absorb. Add the sweet potatoes, diced tomatoes with juices, chicken broth, water, and tomato paste and cook for 3 hours

Dr. Gerard E. Mullin, MD

Dr. Mullin is an associate professor of medicine at The Johns Hopkins Hospital. He is board-certified in internal medicine, gastroenterology, integrative medicine, functional medicine and nutrition. He is an associate editor of several nutrition and integrative medicine journals and the senior editor for the first book for physicians on integrative gastroenterology released by Oxford Press. His latest book, The Gut Balance Revolution (Rodale books, 2015), is the source of these wonderful spice-filled recipes.

Spiced Pork Roast with Cauliflower Mash
Serves 4

Pork loin is a lean, tender cut that makes a perfect weekend roast for a family gathering. Serve leftovers over salad greens or use as a fast no-cook lunch.

Ingredients

2 teaspoons grated fresh ginger
1 teaspoon chili powder, mild or hot
½ teaspoon ground turmeric
2 tablespoons extra-virgin olive oil, divided
1 pound lean pork loin, trimmed of excess fat
½ head cauliflower, cut into florets (about 3 cups florets)
¼ cup chopped cilantro
2 tablespoons wasabi powder or grated fresh horseradish

Directions

Preheat the oven to 400°F.
In a small bowl, place the ginger, chili powder, turmeric, and 1 tablespoon of the oil. Mix well with a spoon or small spatula.
Place the pork in an 11" x 7" baking dish. Spread the oil mixture over the loin and bake, uncovered, for 25 to 30 minutes. Let stand for 5 minutes on a cutting board before slicing.
While the pork is baking, prepare the cauliflower mash. Heat 4 inches

of water in a large pot. Add a steamer basket and insert the florets. Steam for 5 to 6 minutes, or until fork-tender. Transfer to a large bowl and mash with the cilantro, wasabi, or horseradish, and the remaining 1 tablespoon oil. Serve immediately with the pork.

Per serving (1 ½ cups): 213 calories, 26 g protein, 6 g carbohydrates, 10 g total fat, 2 g saturated fat, 74 mg cholesterol, 2 g fiber, 162 mg sodium

Healthy Kitchen Tip: Don't have a steamer basket? Just add the cauliflower florets directly to the pot and steam. Add additional water as needed, ¼ cup at a time.

Ginger Fried Rice
Serves 4

Take-out fried rice isn't only high in MSG, it's also made with white rice that can send your blood sugar skyrocketing. This version has plenty of vegetables and protein that can help anchor your appetite. You'll enjoy the base of brown rice, which is higher in fiber and has a pleasant, chewy texture.

Ingredients

½ cup dry short-grain brown rice
3 tablespoons coconut oil
2 boneless, skinless chicken breasts, cubed, or ½ pound shrimp
1 head bok choy, chopped (about 4 cups)
2 cups frozen shelled edamame
2 tablespoons minced fresh ginger
2 cloves garlic, minced
½ teaspoon Chinese five-spice powder
¼ teaspoon ground turmeric
2 tablespoons reduced sodium, gluten-free soy sauce or tamari sauce (optional)

Directions

Cook the rice according to package directions and set aside.
Heat a large skillet over medium heat. Add the coconut oil. Add the

chicken or shrimp, bok choy, and edamame at once and increase the heat to medium-high. Cook for 3 to 4 minutes, stirring often, or until the chicken and vegetables begin to brown. Add the ginger, garlic, five-spice powder, and turmeric. Cook for 2 to 3 minutes, stirring well, or until the chicken is no longer pink and the juices run clear or the shrimp are opaque. Reduce the heat to medium and stir in the rice and soy or tamari sauce, if using. Serve immediately.

Per serving (1 ½ cups): 376 calories, 28 g protein, 23 g carbohydrates, 16 g total fat, 10 g saturated fat, 54 mg cholesterol, 4 g fiber, 131 mg sodium

Healthy Kitchen Tip: Top with probiotic Pickled Ginger or serve ginger on the side.

Harley Pasternak, M.SC.

As a fitness and nutrition specialist, Pasternak has the largest celebrity clientele roster in the business. Pasternak is also the top selling fitness and diet author in the world whose books include *5-Factor Fitness, 5-Factor Diet, The 5-Factor World Diet, The Body Reset Diet, Body Reset Diet Cookbook,* and his most recent title, *5 Pounds.* He holds a Master of Science in Exercise Physiology and Nutritional Sciences from the University of Toronto and an Honors Degree in Kinesiology from University of Western Ontario.

A Toronto native, he currently resides with his wife and two children in Los Angeles. Whenever I meet with Harley, who is a good friend, we always have to walk as he doesn't believe in seated meetings.

Oven-Baked Swedish Meatballs
Serves 2

Spaghetti and meatballs-Swedish style!

Ingredients

8 ounces extra-lean ground beef

½ small onion, minced
1 egg white
¼ teaspoon Worcestershire sauce
Salt and black pepper
Pinch of ground cinnamon
Pinch of ground cardamom
Pinch of ground allspice
4 ounces whole wheat egg noodles or pasta

Directions

Preheat the oven to 375 degrees F. In a large bowl, combine all the ingredients except the noodles. Using your hands, form small balls. Arrange in a large roasting pan-make sure the meatballs aren't touching-and bake for 15 minutes, turning occasionally to cook on all sides.
Meanwhile, cook the noodles according to the package directions. Drain.
Serve the meatballs atop the noodles.

White Peach Ginger Smoothie
Serves 1

Remember, the riper the fruit, the sweeter the smoothie. If peaches are in season, select the ripest you can find at the market. If not, use frozen peaches.

Serving Tip: Just for fun, the raspberries aren't blended in this drink. Instead, they are dropped into the glass; serve this drink with a spoon for scooping up the berries.

Ingredients

2 peaches, pits removed and chopped
6 ounces fat-free plain Greek yogurt
2 tablespoons fresh lime juice
½ teaspoon finely chopped peeled fresh ginger or pinch of ground ginger
½ cup fresh raspberries

10 de-shelled pistachios, crushed or coarsely chopped (unsalted)

Directions

In a blender or food processor, combine the peaches, yogurt, lime juice, and ginger. Blend until desired consistency. Pour into a tall serving glass. Gently stir in the raspberries and garnish with the pistachios.

Calories: 300, Total Fat: 2 grams, Carbs: 41 grams, Protein: 27 grams, Fiber: 9 grams

Pear Spice Smoothie
Serves 1

This drink is especially good in the fall, when pears are ripe.
Shopping Tip: Experiment with the different types of protein powders now available at the market. Once you've found one you like, you can save money by purchasing a big container.

Ingredients

1 pear, unpeeled, cored and chopped
1 frozen banana, chopped
1 teaspoon finely chopped peeled fresh ginger or pinch of ground ginger
Pinch of ground cinnamon
Pinch of ground nutmeg
2 tablespoons vanilla or unflavored protein powder
½ cup ice cubes or chips

Directions

In a blender or food processor, combine the pear, banana, ginger, cinnamon, nutmeg, protein powder, and ice. Blend until of desired consistency.

Calories: 300, Total Fat: 2 grams, Carbs: 55 grams, Protein: 25 grams
Fiber: 10 grams

Dr. Tom Rifai, MD, FACP and Chef Robert Hindley

Dr. Rifai is a good friend, colleague and fellow physician nutrition specialist. He is the regional medical director of the Henry Ford Metabolic Health program which is based on a time intensive, ultra-individualized and multidisciplinary care lifestyle medicine approach. It includes physician nutrition specialists, registered dietitians, exercise physiologists and trainers as well as behavioral health specialists and – of course Chef Robert Hindley (author of the recipe below)! The ultimate goal is to treat or prevent major metabolic health issues ranging from type 2 diabetes, heart disease, hypertension, cholesterol issues and weight management with a "lifestyle first, medications only where necessary" approach.

This grilled pineapple recipe was created by Chef Rob Hindley who spent 14 years working in several different kitchens with the Ritz Carlton Hotel Company. Before joining Henry Ford Health System 4 years ago, he was the Executive Chef of a high volume Italian restaurant for 12 years. Chef Rob resides in South Lyon Michigan with his wife and three daughters.

Spicy Grilled Pineapple
Serves 4-6

Ingredients

1 fresh pineapple (peeled, cut and cored)
1 teaspoon ground cinnamon
1 teaspoon ground nutmeg
½ teaspoon ground cayenne pepper
2 cups orange juice
2 tablespoons extra virgin olive oil
2 tablespoons balsamic vinegar
1 tablespoon balsamic glaze (store bought works fine or reduce your own balsamic vinegar by ½)

Directions

Cut pineapple, set aside.
Combine remaining ingredients in a small bowl.
Place pineapple rings in a medium casserole dish.
Allow to marinate for 15 minutes to 1 hour.
Grill pineapple slices on medium to high char-broiler or grill.
Turn 2-3 times to create even grill marks, cooking for a total of about 8-10 minutes.
Drizzle with balsamic glaze and serve.

Chef Michael Schley

Chef Michael, who also happens to be my brother-in-law, started his culinary career working at Gardens on Glendon and Kate Mantilini in Beverly Hills, CA hosting many of LA's movie Premier parties. He then moved to San Francisco where he attended the California Culinary Academy. During this time, he earned an exclusive externship studying under the legendary Michelin starred chef Thomas Keller at his world renowned restaurant, The French Laundry, in Yountville, CA. Upon completion of his externship, he worked at famous restaurants, Aqua & Plumpjack Café in San Francisco, CA. He now resides in San Mateo, CA with his wife and two young boys and runs a successful catering business called Umami Togo. He integrates a lot of spices in his daily cooking and tries to keep it "spicy" at home. One of his favorite spices is cumin because a small amount packs a lot of flavor & it's quite versatile. His boys, Colten and Dylan, put cinnamon on almost everything (and they don't even know it's good for them).

"Tagine" Style Chicken, Beef or Eggplant
Serves 4-6

Historically Tagine is a succulent stew made of meats and vegetables and traditionally cooked in a conical clay pot to allow the steam to rise, condense and drip back down to the stew. The traditional method of cooking is to place the tagine over coals, and typically the dish includes meat, chicken or fish, and most often vegetables or fruit.

Ingredients

(2 each medium eggplant diced into 2 inch pieces) or
(1.5 pounds of diced beef stew meat cut into 1-2 inch pieces) or
4 each boneless & skinless chicken thighs cut into 1 inch dice
1 each medium yellow onion diced into 1 inch pieces
3 each garlic clove minced
1 tbs minced ginger (if you like ginger add more)
½ cup pitted kalamata olives chopped
½ bunch flat leaf parsley chopped
½ bunch cilantro chopped
1 tsp turmeric
¼ water or chicken stock
Olive Oil

Directions

Have all your things in place. Start with a stock pot or soup pot.
Heat oil on medium high for a minute.
When hot, add onion and let brown for roughly 3 minutes or until caramelization is achieved.
Next, add chicken, eggplant or beef and cook another 3 minutes.
Finally, add the turmeric, ginger and garlic and reduce to medium heat for about 3 minutes stirring occasionally.*
*For additional flavor: Add 10oz can diced tomato, 1 can coconut milk, orange zest and juice of 1 orange & ¼ tsp cinnamon.
Then add the olives and the water or stock, cilantro and parsley (*and other items if using, the fun things with recipes is that they are a template for you to make it yours) cover with lid and simmer for 30 minutes until chicken is tender.

Barry Sears Ph.D.

Barry Sears Ph.D. is the author of #1 New York Times best-seller *The Zone* that started the field of anti-inflammatory nutrition in 1995. He has sold more than 6 million copies of his various books on the application of his Zone technology, and these books have been translated into 22 different languages. He has also published more than 40 scientific articles and has 14 U.S. Patents in the areas of drug delivery technology and the dietary modulation of hormones to reduce inflammatory responses. He is currently the President of the non-profit Inflammation Research Foundation. I met Barry while filming my TV show Fit TV's Diet Doctor and we have stayed in touch ever since and I frequently email him questions about anti-inflammatory nutrition. Here is how he incorporates spices into his diet.

From Barry: "Here is my standard carbohydrate part of most of my dinner at home."

Dr. Sears Vegetable Spice Medley

Ingredients

2 red peppers
1 red onion
6 garlic cloves
6 oz. grape tomatoes
6 oz. of mixed broccoli and cauliflower florets
1 pound of asparagus
4 oz. mushrooms

Directions

I will puree these in a food processor and then cook them for 20 minutes in a T-Fal Actifry (low heat at 375 F provided by circulating hot air and moving arm to stir the vegetables). I will take the vegetables out after cooking and a the following spices using about three shakes of each:

Mustard	Cardamom
Coriander	Basil
Crushed rosemary	Cilantro
Toasted sesame seed	Tarragon
Oregano	Turmeric
Thyme	Curry
Marjoram	Cumin

I will put this total mixture in a soup pot and add some chicken broth and slowly simmer. I will use half for dinner and save the other half for the next day. Then I add about 3-4 oz. of low-fat protein plus some extra virgin olive to complete the meal.

Dr. Travis Stork, MD

Dr. Travis Stork is an Emmy®-nominated host of the award-winning talk show *The Doctors*, and an emergency medicine physician. He graduated Magna Cum Laude from Duke University as a member of Phi Beta Kappa and earned his M.D. with honors from the University of Virginia, being elected into the prestigious honor society of Alpha Omega Alpha for outstanding academic achievement. Based on his experiences as an ER physician, Dr. Stork is passionate about teaching people simple methods to prevent illness before it happens with the goal of maximizing the enjoyment of a healthy life. He is a New York Times #1 bestselling author of *The Lose Your Belly Diet – Change Your Gut, Change Your Life, The Doctor's Diet, The Doctor's Diet Cookbook, The Lean Belly Prescription, and The Doctor Is In: A 7-Step Prescription for Optimal Wellness.*

Having worked with him dozens of times on *The Doctors*, I can tell you firsthand that Dr. Travis is the real deal - very intelligent and also incredibly kind and caring. He lives in the Nashville area and his hobbies include mountain biking, kayaking, and spending time outdoors.

Dr. Travis puts Chow-Chows on his veggie burgers as a condiment and on bean based chips with some grated cheese and beans to add flavor to his homemade nachos.

Mediterranean Chow-Chow (Recipe from *The Lose Your Belly Diet,* Ghost Mountain Books, 2016)

Chow-chow is a type of relish that is popular in the South, Midwest and Canada. They are traditionally made from bountiful vegetable gardens and preserved or canned for the winter months. They can contain a wide range of veggies and served as a condiment or side dish. Some were pickled and many contained huge amounts of sugar. Travis has recipes that are friendlier to the gut microbiome, his Little Buddies, filled with raw veggies to support the gut microbiome and without the sugar. "The Lose Your Belly Diet" Chow-chow recipes feature fresh herbs, savory spices, citrus and all kinds of raw veggies. Fiber-rich you can add them to salads, put on burritos/tacos or top sandwiches, burgers, omelets, etc. There is a Mediterranean recipe, South-of-the-Border or Coleslaw version.

Ingredients

4 cups Mediterranean vegetables, diced into 1/2 inch pieces (any combo of tomatoes, garlic, onions, zucchini, fennel, mushrooms, green beans, asparagus, e.g.)
1 Tbsp extra-virgin olive oil
1 Tbsp balsamic vinegar
1 tsp lemon juice
1/8 tsp salt
Freshly ground pepper
1 Tbsp fresh basil, chopped
1 Tbsp fresh oregano, chopped

Directions

Place all ingredients in a large bowl. Cover and store in the fridge. Optional: Make it a light meal by adding 1 oz cubed mozzarella and 10 large black olives, chopped. Adds some good fats!

Chef Neal Swidler

Neal Swidler, who also happens to be my cousin, is the Executive Chef of the iconic Broussard's Restaurant in the French Quarter. Chef Neal has 20 years of experience in Executive Level Restaurant Management and Concept Development. He spent many years in some of the best kitchens in New Orleans, including Chef Emeril Lagasse's Delmonico and Nola Restaurant, as well as Chef Mike Fennely's Mike's on the Avenue. Chef Neal also specialized in unique startup and multiunit concepts serving as corporate Chef for the JFB Corporation, which owns Juan's Flying Burrito and Slice Restaurants, before opening his own original concept, Lucky Rooster. Lucky Rooster was awarded New Orleans best Asian Mashup Restaurant in 2013, within six months of opening. Originally from Chicago, Chef Neal graduated from the University of Arizona, then attended the prestigious Culinary Institute of America in Hyde Park, New York where he graduated at the top of his class with Honors. Chef Neal resides in New Orleans and owns Popstars Icicle Treats with his three teenage daughters.

Maque Choux
Serves 8

Ingredients

8 Ears of Corn
1 Jalapeno Pepper, diced
2 cups Celery, diced
2 cups Green Bell Pepper, diced
1 qt. Onions, diced
2 Tbl Minced Garlic
1 Tbl Creole Seasoning
2 Tbl Worcestershire Sauce
2 Tbl Crystal Hot Sauce

Directions

Place the Ears of Corn on a sheet tray and roast them for 30 minutes in a 300 degree oven. Once they are cooked remove them from the oven and let them cool to room temperature.
Once the Ears are cool enough to handle remove the husks and silk, then cut the kernels from the cob and set them aside.

In a large sauté pan over medium heat "sweat" the Onions, Peppers, Celery and Garlic with the Creole Seasoning until they are translucent.
Next deglaze the pan with the Hot Sauce and Worcestershire and allow the liquid in the pan to reduce until it is almost dry.
When the liquid had reduced enough add the Corn to the sauté pan and toss to combine.
Lay the mix evenly onto sheet trays and chill the mix in the refrigerator.

Chef Neal's Famous Creole Seasoning

Ingredients

6 ½ tsp Korean chili powder
4 ½ tsp paprika
½ tsp garlic powder
1 tsp dried thyme
1 ½ tsp kosher salt
¼ tsp black pepper
¾ tsp dried oregano
½ tsp celery salt
¼ tsp cayenne pepper

Directions

Mix all together and store in an air tight container.

Chuck Wagner

Chuck Wagner has been a good friend for over a decade and makes one of my favorite Napa Cabernets. Chuck, the owner and winemaker of Caymus Vineyards, was born in Rutherford, Napa Valley, into a family of farmers with deep roots in the region. He was just 19 when he started Caymus with his parents, and the Wagners became famed for their Cabernet Sauvignon. Still a farmer at heart, Chuck believes in enjoying the simple pleasures of life. This Brazilian chicken recipe is a great pairing with Caymus Cabernet – untraditional and an exceptional way to showcase the flavors of both the food and the wine.

Brazilian-Style Grilled Chicken with Chimichurri
Serves 4-6

For the Chimichurri:
2 c Parsley, washed and picked
1 c Cilantro, washed and picked
½ c Oregano, washed and picked
2 ea Garlic Cloves
½ c Extra Virgin Olive Oil
¼ ea Small Jalapeno, optional
¼ c Red Wine Vinegar
to taste Salt and Pepper

Directions: In a food processor, add all ingredients and puree the mixture until smooth. Season with salt and pepper. Keep cold until ready to serve.

For the Chicken:
1 ea Whole Chicken, approximately 1½-2 pounds
2 T Sea Salt, coarsely ground
4 ea Garlic Cloves
4 T Olive Oil, extra virgin
1 T Rosemary, fresh, chopped
1 T Cumin, toasted and ground
1 T Fennel Seed, toasted and ground

1 T Sweet Paprika
¼ t White Pepper, ground
As needed Mesquite or hardwood-based charcoal

In a food processor, process the garlic and olive oil to make a paste. Season the chicken with, rosemary, cumin, fennel, sweet paprika and white pepper. Pour the garlic and olive oil mixture over chicken halves, turning chicken to coat both sides. Rub all sides of the chicken with the oil and spices. Refrigerate covered overnight.

Build a fire with the charcoal. Allow the fire to cool quite a bit; it is important to grill the chicken over a medium to low fire as it will take some time to cook and the slower the chicken cooks the more tender and juicy the result will be. Plan on 15-20 minutes per side. After grilling, allow the chicken to rest for approximately ten minutes before serving. Place the chicken on a serving platter and serve with the chimichurri.

Dr. Jennifer Warren, MD

Dr. Warren is the co-founder and Medical Director of Physicians Healthy Weight Center based in North Hampton, NH. Dr. Warren is a graduate of Tufts University School of Medicine, and is board-certified by the American Board of Obesity Medicine, and the American Board of Family Medicine. She recommends the regular use of spices in cooking to her patients, for both flavor and health benefits, and frequently sneaks extra spices into her husband's cooking when he's not looking. Dr. Warren is a trusted colleague and friend and we speak by phone frequently. She brought in her team to help me with several recipes for this book.

Melissa Ransdell is a nutrition and lifestyle educator at Physicians Healthy Weight Center. She works part time at PHWC, while studying full time-time as student at the University of New Hampshire, studying Dietetics. She teaches salsa dancing, wrote the Turmeric Latte Recipe, and enjoys both often.

Amy Buzzell is a nutrition and lifestyle educator at Physicians Healthy Weight Center. Amy has a Bachelor of Science degree in in Nutrition Science from the University of New Hampshire, and an M.S. in Clinical Nutrition from the New York Institute of Technology. She enjoys cinnamon in her coffee, creating new recipes, and modifying old favorites to make them healthier.

Turmeric Latte
Serves 1

Ingredients

1 cup coconut milk
1 tsp Vanilla extract
2 packets Stevia
½ tsp Turmeric
¼ tsp Ginger
¼ tsp Cinnamon
Desired amount of Espresso or black coffee
Directions

Heat coconut milk, vanilla extract, stevia, turmeric, ginger and cinnamon in a saucepan and heat until warm. Remove from heat and add milk mixture to espresso or black coffee.

Cinnamon Almond Coffee

Add ¼ tsp Cinnamon in Coffee with unsweetened vanilla almond milk and a sweetener of your choice for a spiced up morning coffee!

Tomato Curry Soup
Serves 4

Ingredients

1 can of crushed tomatoes, undrained

1 medium onion, finely diced
1 green chili pepper with seeds removed, finely diced
2 cloves of crushed garlic
1 tbs tomato paste
4 cups of low sodium organic vegetable broth
½ tsp organic curry powder
2 tbsp extra virgin olive oil

Directions

In a large pan, heat oil over medium heat, then sauté onion, chili and garlic until soft. Add the can of crushed tomatoes to the saucepan and mix with the sauted vegetables. Cook for 5 minutes; stir often. In a separate bowl mix the tomato paste, vegetable broth, and curry powder. Pour mixture into saucepan, blend, then simmer for 7-10 minutes. Serve and enjoy!

Super Simple Spicy Soups
Serves 4

Sometimes making a homemade soup is time consuming and difficult to get right. Try convenient resealable 'boxes of soup' by Pacific Organic, Imagine, or Trader Joe's (flavors include Sweet Potato, Butternut Squash, Pumpkin, Tomato, Ginger Carrot, etc.) Choose low sodium and organic versions. Make these special by adding spices, and protein, using the recipes below.

Quick Spiced Tomato Soup
Serves 4

Ingredients

Pre-made tomato soup (popular brands: Trader Joe's, Imagine, Pacific Organic)
½ tsp curry powder (or to taste)
1 tsp Olive oil

Directions

Mix curry powder in a bowl with olive oil to evenly disperse the spice. Add the curry-oil mixture to a pre-made tomato soup. Top with ½ cup of Fat-free Kraft Shredded Mozzarella Cheese, 1 ounce 75% fat-free Cabot Cheddar, or ½ cup fat-free feta for protein, then heat in microwave to melt - simple and delicious!

Quick Spiced Winter Soups
Serves 4

Pick your favorite: pre-made soup: Sweet potato, carrot, squash or pumpkin work best.

Ingredients

1 tsp Olive oil
Choice of spices:
½ tsp curry (or to taste)
½ tsp ginger (or to taste)
½ tsp cinnamon (or to taste)

Directions

Time to get creative! Mix spices in a bowl with olive oil to evenly disperse the spice. Add the spice-oil mixture to a pre-made winter vegetable soup.

Favorite combinations: Cinnamon-Sweet potato, Ginger-Squash, Curry-Carrot, Cinnamon-Pumpkin. Heat, add and enjoy!

Quick Tip To Add Protein: Top soup with fat free or reduced fat cheeses or add diced chicken.

Dr. Bojana Jankovic Weatherly, MD

Dr. Bojana is a board-certified internal medicine physician with an interest in integrative medicine, nutrition and mindfulness. She is an educator, speaker and author and her videos and articles on health and wellness can be found on drbojana.com. She serves as the Chief Medical Officer of WellStart Health, a mobile platform that helps prevent and reverse chronic disease by health coaching and empowering people to make healthy lifestyle choices. She relocated to NYC from LA this year where she lives with her husband and two young children. Bojana and I met last year through a mutual friend and I have enjoyed getting to know her and seeing her progress in her integrative medicine and nutrition career.

Black Bean Brownies
Yields 12 brownies

Ingredients

1 can black beans (drained and well rinsed) – 1.5 cups
3 table spoons cocoa powder
½ cup rolled old fashion oats
½ teaspoon baking powder
2 table spoons coarsely ground flax seeds
¼ teaspoon ground nutmeg
1 teaspoon organic ground cinnamon
¼ cup olive oil
½ cup maple syrup
1/8 cup soy milk
2 teaspoons pure vanilla extract
2/3 cup finely cut walnuts
2/3 cup dark chocolate chips

Directions

Preheat oven to 350 F.
After rinsing and draining the canned beans, place them on stove top at medium heat. Mix frequently, ensuring they don't stick to the pan,

and cook until they soften up enough so they can be easily mashed up.

In a separate bowl, mix cocoa powder, oats, baking powder, flax seeds, nutmeg and cinnamon.

Add wet ingredients: olive oil, maple syrup, soy milk and vanilla extract, and mix well.

Add black beans and mix well.

Put the mixture in a blender or a food processor and blend well.

Put the blended mixture in a bowl, add chocolate chips and finely chopped walnuts, and gently mix.

Grease the pan with olive oil or vegetable oil spray.

Pour the mixture into the pan.

Cook the brownies for 20 minutes, then let them cool down for 10-15 minutes, before cutting and serving them.

Lentil Soup
Serves 6

Ingredients

*note: All (or as many as possible) of my ingredients are organic.
2 cups dry lentils
½ cup spinach
5-10 cherry tomatoes
5 cups water (note: you may wish to modify slightly to your taste and desirable consistency)
1-2 cups vegetable broth (note: you may wish to modify slightly to your taste and desirable consistency)
1.5 medium to large carrots
½-1 bell pepper
¼ tsp cardamom
1 tsp dried basil
¼ tsp coriander
¼ tsp salt (or to taste)
extra virgin olive oil
½ cup chopped onion

Directions

In a large pot, heat extra virgin olive oil on medium heat.
Add chopped onions and cook, while stirring, for 1 minute.
Add chopped bell peppers and chopped carrots.
Stir for a few minutes and add a little water or vegetable broth, as needed.
Add dry lentils, followed by the rest of the water and vegetable broth.
Add chopped spinach and cherry tomato slices.
Continue stirring and bring to a boil.
Add cardamom, dried basil, coriander and salt and mix well.
Reduce the heat and simmer for 1 hour, or longer, if needed.

Deborah Parker Wong, DWSET

Deborah Parker Wong, DWSET is Global Wine Editor for SOMM Journal, The Tasting and Clever Root magazines where she reports on the wine and spirits industries with an emphasis on trends. In addition, she contributes features on business and production technology to Spirited magazine. Deborah co-authored "1000 Great Everyday Wines" published by Dorling Kindersley in 2011.

Deborah holds a Diploma from the London-based Wine & Spirit Education Trust, she teaches WSET certification courses and as an adjunct professor in the wine studies program at Santa Rosa Junior College. In addition to writing and speaking about wine, Deborah provides high-level consulting services to the trade, judges wine competitions and scores wine for Planet Grape Wine Review. Her motto is: To learn, read. To know, write. To master, teach.
Favorite spice-laden dishes and wine pairings

Haydari – Turkish Yogurt Dip
Serves 8

If you enjoy Indian raita or Persian mastokhiar, this thick, tangy spread is right up your alley.

Ingredients

1 1/2 cups strained yogurt (or Greek style thick yogurt)
3 Tbs feta cheese, grated
2 Tbs fresh dill, finely chopped
1 Tbs fresh mint, finely chopped
1 Tbs fresh fennel fronds, finely chopped
1/3 c walnuts, finely chopped
1 Tbs lemon juice
1-2 cloves garlic, pressed
Salt to taste
1 Tbs olive oil for garnish
1 tsp sumac or paprika for garnish

Directions

Mix all the ingredients until blended thoroughly. Refrigerate until ready to serve.

Wine pairing: Wine and yogurt pairings can be tricky but there are two wines that fit the bill. Chablis which is made from unoaked Chardonnay has high acidity and is often described as having yogurty flavors from undergoing malolactic fermentation. Verdicchio is a high-acid Italian white grape variety that has citrus, almond and fennel notes. This wine ideally mirrors the acidity, herbs and nuts found in the dish.

DEBORAH PARKER WONG'S SPICE AND WINE PAIRINGS

Spice	White and Red Wines
Turmeric and Curry	Riesling, Torrontes, aged Semillion
Cinnamon	Pinot Noir, Grenache, aged Rioja (Tempranillo)
Ginger	Chenin Blanc, Gewurztraminer, Pinot Gris
Cumin	Chardonnay, Barolo (Nebbiolo)
Cayenne	Champagne, sparkling wine, Lambrusco
Oregano	Sangiovese, Douro dry reds, Cabernet Franc, Carmenere
Basil and Pesto	Sauvignon Blanc, Gruner Veltiner, Soave (Garganega), Verdicchio, rosé
Cilantro and Coriander	Sauvignon Blanc, Beaujolais (Gamay), Grenache
Thyme	Cabernet Sauvignon, Sangiovese, Pinotage
Rosemary and Herbs de Provence	GSM (Grenache, Syrah, Mourvedre), Malbec, Zinfandel
Nutmeg and Baking spice	Pinot Noir, Carignan, aged Chianti (Sangiovese)
Cardamom	Viognier, Bordeaux Blends, Cabernet Franc, Carmenere
Black pepper	Pinot Noir, Cabernet Sauvignon, Valpolicella (red blend)
Star anise and Chinese Five Spice	Pinot Noir, Barbera, Syrah

Dr. Adrienne Youdim, MD FACP

Dr. Youdim specializes in medical weight loss and nutritional therapy. She is currently Associate Professor of Medicine at UCLA School of Medicine and Cedars-Sinai Medical Center. In addition to her clinical practice, Dr. Youdim lectures extensively and has appeared on local and national news and television programs. She is a mother of 3 children ages 13, 10 and 4 and in her free time she loves running, entertaining and watching Chopped. dradrienneyoudim.com

Working Moms 10-Minute Chicken
Serves 4

Ingredients

1 pound chicken breast tenders
1/2 lemon
1/2 tsp salt
1/2 tsp ground pepper
2 sprigs fresh thyme (1 tsp)
1 sprig fresh rosemary (1 tsp)
1 TBs extra virgin olive oil

Directions

Put all ingredients in a large ziplock and mix. Refrigerate for at least 30 minutes. (Preparation can be left over night as well)
Use a grill plate over the stove top. Turn to medium to medium/high heat. When warm spray plate with olive oil spray. Place marinated chicken tenders on grill plate for approximately 3-4 minutes per side. Use a fork or knife to poke center - juice should run clear when ready.

Optional side
1 cup red or white quinoa
2 cups water
1/2 tsp salt
2 tomatoes on the vine
3 Persian cucumbers
1 small bunch cilantro

Directions

In a separate pot bring quinoa and two cups water to a boil then reduce to simmer. Simmer slowly for approximately 20 minutes until liquid has evaporated. Remove from stove to cool.
Dice tomatoes into 1 cm cubes (approximately)
Dice cucumbers to 1 cm cubes (approximately) (no need to peel)
Finely chop one bunch cilantro leaves
Mix tomato and cucumbers with quinoa once cool
Mix in 1/2 tsp. salt and 1/2 squeezed lemon juice.
Toss and serve alongside chicken tenders

CONCLUSION

Before writing this book, I was intrigued by the potential health benefits and healing power of spices but I knew very little about their history. Through the process of writing this book, not only am I amazed by the rich and fascinating history of spices, I'm even more excited than ever to integrate them into my diet as much as possible and I hope you are too.

One of the most wonderful aspects of working on this book was sharing my enthusiasm for spices with my friends and colleagues and finding that many of them were equally as excited about the health benefits of spices. The best part was their eagerness to share their favorite spice recipes in this book. Another exciting part of writing this book is that I've pledged to give 100% of the profits to Action Against Hunger, one of the leading organizations fighting childhood malnutrition globally. So by purchasing this book, you are not only improving your health, you are potentially improving the health of children suffering from malnutrition and starvation around the world.

I hope this book is just the beginning of your lifelong journey exploring spices and that in addition to the suggestions in this book, you find new and wonderful ways of including spices into your diet to improve your health. In addition, if you need to lose weight, I'm confident that spices can help you do that too—they don't work magically by themselves, but when combined with a healthy diet, stress management, adequate sleep, and regular exercise, they can almost certainly help. And no matter what diet you follow, your food will definitely taste better and will be even healthier.

I'm going to continue following all the latest research on spices as well as continuing to work on adding more spices into my diet, and I plan share all my insights, tips and recipes on facebook throughout my ongoing journey. I hope that you will do the same—I love to hear from readers, and who knows, I may include one of your recipes or tips in my next book.

In good health,

Melina B. Jampolis, MD

Facebook.com/drmelina

Twitter: @drmelina

PERSONAL SPICE NOTES

REFERENCES

AAPS J (2013) 15: 195. Gupta, Subash C., et al. "Therapeutic Roles of Curcumin: Lessons Learned from Clinical Trials." *SpringerLink*, Springer US, 10 Nov. 2012, link.springer.com/article/10.1208%2Fs12248-012-9432-8.

"CDC Features." *Centers for Disease Control and Prevention*, Centers for Disease Control and Prevention, 4 Mar. 2016, www.cdc.gov/features/sodium/index.html.

Lv, Jun, et al. "Consumption of Spicy Foods and Total and Cause Specific Mortality: Population Based Cohort Study." *BMJ*, British Medical Journal Publishing Group, 4 Aug. 2015, www.bmj.com/content/351/bmj.h3942.

Star Spices

Cinnamon

"1 Daily Teaspoon Of This Spice Will Transform Your Life." *Healthy and Natural World*, 10 Nov. 2016, www.healthyandnaturalworld.com/how to-use-cinnamon-as-a-medicine.

Filippone, Peggy Trowbridge. "Interesting Highlights in the Colorful History of Cinnamon." *The Spruce*, www.thespruce.com/history-of-cinnamon-1807584.

Morgenstern, Kat. "Cinnamon (Cinnamomum Zeylanicum Blume)

Lauracaeae." *Cinnamon (Cinnamomum Zeylanicum) - History and Uses - Sacred Earth Ethnobotany Resources*, www.sacredearth.com/ethnobotany/plantprofiles/cinnamon.php.

Allen, R.W.; Schwartzman, E.; Baker, W.L.; Coleman, C.I.; Phung, O.J. Cinnamon Use in Type 2 Diabetes: An Updated Systematic Review and Meta-Analysis. The Annals of Family Medicine 2013, 11, 452-459.

Davis, P.A.; Yokoyama, W. Cinnamon intake lowers fasting blood glucose: meta-analysis. Journal of medicinal food 2011, 14, 884-889.

Akilen, R.; Tsiami, A.; Devendra, D.; Robinson, N. Cinnamon in glycaemic control: Systematic review and meta analysis. Clinical Nutrition 2012, 31, 609-615.
Leach, M.J.; Kumar, S. Cinnamon for diabetes mellitus. The Cochrane Library 2012.

Akilen, R.; Pimlott, Z.; Tsiami, A.; Robinson, N. Effect of short-term administration of cinnamon on blood pressure in patients with prediabetes and type 2 diabetes. Nutrition 2013, 29, 1192-1196.

Jungbauer, A.; Medjakovic, S. Anti-inflammatory properties of culinary herbs and spices that ameliorate the effects of metabolic syndrome. Maturitas 2012, 71, 227-239.

Wahlqvist, M.L.; Lee, M.-S.; Lee, J.-T.; Hsu, C.-C.; Chou, Y.-C.; Fang, W.-H.; Liu, H.-Y.; Xiu, L.; Andrews, Z.B. Cinnamon users with prediabetes have a better fasting working memory: a cross-sectional function study. Nutrition Research 2016, 36, 305-310.

Azimi, P.; Ghiasvand, R.; Feizi, A.; Hariri, M.; Abbasi, B. Effects of Cinnamon, Cardamom, Saffron, and Ginger Consumption on Markers of Glycemic Control, Lipid Profile, Oxidative Stress, and Inflammation in Type 2 Diabetes Patients. The review of diabetic studies: RDS 2013, 11, 258-266.

Turmeric

"6 Reasons Why To-Be Bride And Groom Have A Haldi Ceremony Before Their Wedding." Edited by Team BollywoodShaadis, *BollywoodShaadis*, Mar. 2017, www.bollywoodshaadis.com/articles/significance-of-haldi-ceremony-in-indian-weddings-3198.
Avey, Tori. "What Is the History of Turmeric?" *PBS*, Public Broadcasting

Service, 9 Mar. 2015, www.pbs.org/food/the-history-kitchen/turmeric-history/.

Aggarwal, B. B., & Yost, D. (2011). Healing spices: how to use 50 everyday and exotic spices to boost health and beat disease. New York: Sterling Pub. Co.

Sahebkar, A. Are Curcuminoids Effective C-Reactive Protein-Lowering Agents in Clinical Practice? Evidence from a Meta-Analysis. Phytotherapy Research 2014, 28, 633-642.

Derosa, G.; Maffioli, P.; Simental-Mendia, L.E.; Bo, S.; Sahebkar, A. Effect of curcumin on circulating interleukin-6 concentrations: A systematic review and meta-analysis of randomized controlled trials. Pharmacol Res 2016, 111, 394-404.

Sahebkar, A. A systematic review and meta-analysis of randomized controlled trials investigating the effects of curcumin on blood lipid levels. Clinical Nutrition 2014, 33, 406-414.

Chuengsamarn, S.; Rattanamongkolgul, S.; Luechapudiporn, R.; Phisalaphong, C.; Jirawatnotai, S. Curcumin Extract for Prevention of Type 2 Diabetes. Diabetes Care 2012, 35, 2121-2127.

Akazawa, N.; Choi, Y.; Miyaki, A.; Tanabe, Y.; Sugawara, J.; Ajisaka, R.; Maeda, S. Curcumin ingestion and exercise training improve vascular endothelial function in postmenopausal women. Nutrition Research 2012, 32, 795-799.

Akazawa, N.; Choi, Y.; Miyaki, A.; Tanabe, Y.; Sugawara, J.; Ajisaka, R.; Maeda, S. Effects of curcumin intake and aerobic exercise training on arterial compliance in postmenopausal women. Artery Research 2013, 7, 67-72.

Chuengsamarn, S.; Rattanamongkolgul, S.; Phonrat, B.; Tungtrongchitr, R.; Jirawatnotai, S. Reduction of atherogenic risk in patients with type 2 diabetes by curcuminoid extract: a randomized controlled trial. The Journal of Nutritional Biochemistry 2014, 25, 144-150.

Na, L.X.; Li, Y.; Pan, H.Z.; Zhou, X.L.; Sun, D.J.; Meng, M.; Li, X.X.; Sun, C.H. Curcuminoids exert glucose-lowering effect in type 2 diabetes by decreasing serum free fatty acids: a double-blind, placebo-controlled trial. Molecular nutrition & food research 2013, 57, 1569-1577.

Tang, M.; Larson-Meyer, D.E.; Liebman, M. Effect of cinnamon and turmeric on urinary oxalate excretion, plasma lipids, and plasma glucose in healthy subjects. The American Journal of Clinical Nutrition 2008, 87, 1262-1267.

Wickenberg, J.; Ingemansson, S.L.; Hlebowicz, J. Effects of Curcuma longa (turmeric) on postprandial plasma glucose and insulin in healthy subjects. Nutrition Journal 2010, 9, 1-5.

Daily, J.W.; Yang, M.; Park, S. Efficacy of Turmeric Extracts and Curcumin for Alleviating the Symptoms of Joint Arthritis: A Systematic Review and Meta-Analysis of Randomized Clinical Trials. J Med Food 2016, 19, 717-729.

Al-Karawi, D.; Al Mamoori, D.A.; Tayyar, Y. The Role of Curcumin Administration in Patients with Major Depressive Disorder: Mini Meta-Analysis of Clinical Trials. Phytother Res 2016, 30, 175-183.

Mazzanti, G.; Di Giacomo, S. Curcumin and Resveratrol in the Management of Cognitive Disorders: What is the Clinical Evidence? Molecules 2016, 21, 1243.

Ng, T.P.; Chiam, P.C.; Lee, T.; Chua, H.C.; Lim, L.; Kua, E.H. Curry consumption and cognitive function in the elderly. Am J Epidemiol 2006, 164, 898-906.

Darvesh, A.S.; Carroll, R.T.; Bishayee, A.; Geldenhuys, W.J.; Van der Schyf, C.J. Oxidative stress and Alzheimer's disease: dietary polyphenols as potential therapeutic agents. Expert Review of Neurotherapeutics 2010, 10, 729-745.

Hugel, H.M. Brain Food for Alzheimer-Free Ageing: Focus on Herbal Medicines. Adv Exp Med Biol 2015, 863, 95-116.

Patcharatrakul, T.; Gonlachanvit, S. Chili Peppers, Curcumins, and Prebiotics in Gastrointestinal Health and Disease. Current Gastroenterology Reports 2016, 18, 19.

Craig, W.J. Health-promoting properties of common herbs. The American Journal of Clinical Nutrition 1999, 70, 491s-499s.

Ginger

Nichol, C. (2015). Essential spices and herbs: discover them, understand them, enjoy them. Berkeley, CA: Rockridge Press.

says, J, and Nana Esi says. "How Ginger Is Used In Traditional & Modern Medicine » The Candida Diet." *The Candida Diet*, 12 Jan. 2017, www.thecandidadiet.com/ginger-traditional-and-modern-medicine/.

Bode, Ann M. "The Amazing and Mighty Ginger." *Herbal Medicine: Biomolecular and Clinical Aspects. 2nd Edition.*, U.S. National Library of Medicine, 1 Jan. 1970.

Arablou, T.; Aryaeian, N.; Valizadeh, M.; Sharifi, F.; Hosseini, A.; Djalali, M. The effect of ginger consumption on glycemic status, lipid profile and some inflammatory markers in patients with type 2 diabetes mellitus.

International journal of food sciences and nutrition 2014, 65, 515-520. Mahluji, S.; Attari, V.E.; Mobasseri, M.; Payahoo, L.; Ostadrahimi, A.; Golzari, S.E.J. Effects of ginger (Zingiber officinale) on plasma glucose level, HbA1c and insulin sensitivity in type 2 diabetic patients. International journal of food sciences and nutrition 2013, 64, 682-686.

Mazidi, M.; Gao, H.K.; Rezaie, P.; Ferns, G.A. The effect of ginger supplementation on serum C-reactive protein, lipid profile and glycaemia: a systematic review and meta analysis. Food Nutr Res 2016, 60, 32613.

Imani, H.; Tabibi, H.; Najafi, I.; Atabak, S.; Hedayati, M.; Rahmani, L. Effects of ginger on serum glucose, advanced glycation end products, and inflammation in peritoneal dialysis patients. Nutrition 2015, 31, 703-707.

Mozaffari-Khosravi, H.; Talaei, B.; Jalali, B.A.; Najarzadeh, A.; Mozayan, M.R. The effect of ginger powder supplementation on insulin resistance and glycemic indices in patients with type 2 diabetes: a randomized, double-blind, placebo-controlled trial. Complement Ther Med 2014, 22, 9-16.

Shidfar, F.; Rajab, A.; Rahideh, T.; Khandouzi, N.; Hosseini, S.; Shidfar, S. The effect of ginger (Zingiber officinale) on glycemic markers in patients with type 2 diabetes. Journal of Complementary and Integrative Medicine 2015, 12, 165-170.
Bartels, E.M.; Folmer, V.N.; Bliddal, H.; Altman, R.D.; Juhl, C.; Tarp, S.; Zhang, W.; Christensen, R. Efficacy and safety of ginger in osteoarthritis patients: a meta-analysis of randomized placebo-controlled trials.

Osteoarthritis and Cartilage 2015, 23, 13-21.

Palatty, P.L.; Haniadka, R.; Valder, B.; Arora, R.; Baliga, M.S. Ginger in the prevention of nausea and vomiting: a review. Crit Rev Food Sci Nutr 2013, 53, 659-669.

Saenghong, N.; Wattanathorn, J.; Muchimapura, S.; Tongun, T.; Piyavhatkul, N.; Banchonglikitkul, C.; Kajsongkram, T. Zingiber officinale Improves Cognitive Function of the Middle-Aged Healthy Women. Evidence-Based Complementary and Alternative Medicine 2012, 2012, 9.

Cayenne Pepper

Chapman, Kristin, and Julia Bianco. "Capsaicin - Neurobiology Of Disease 07." *Google Sites*, Connecticut College, sites.google.com/a/conncoll.edu/neurobiology-of-disease-07/home/capsaicin.

Legacy, Herbal. "A History of the Healing Chili." *Cayenne History*, www.herballegacy.com/Cayenne_History.html.

"Cayenne Pepper." The Epicentre, theepicentre.com/spice/cayenne-pepper/.

Whiting, S.; Derbyshire, E.; Tiwari, B.K. Capsaicinoids and capsinoids. A potential role for weight management? A systematic review of the evidence. Appetite 2012, 59, 341-348.

Zheng, J.; Zheng, S.; Feng, Q.; Zhang, Q.; Xiao, X. Dietary capsaicin and its anti-obesity potency: from mechanism to clinical implications. Bioscience Reports 2017, 37.

Srinivasan, K. Biological Activities of Red Pepper (Capsicum annuum) and Its Pungent Principle Capsaicin: A Review. Crit Rev Food Sci Nutr 2016, 56, 1488-1500.

Oregano

"The History of Oregano | MySpicer.com | Spices, Herbs & Seasonings." MySpicer | Spices, Herbs, Seasonings, 10 Jan. 2014,
Nurmi, A.; Mursu, J.; Nurmi, T.; Nyyssönen, K.; Alfthan, G.; Hiltunen, R.; Kaikkonen, J.; Salonen, J.T.; Voutilainen, S. Consumption of Juice Fortified with Oregano Extract Markedly Increases Excretion of Phenolic Acids but

Lacks Short- and Long-Term Effects on Lipid Peroxidation in Healthy Nonsmoking Men. Journal of Agricultural and Food Chemistry 2006, 54, 5790-5796.

Özdemir, B.; Ekbul, A.; Topal, N.; Sarandöl, E.; Sağ, S.; Başer, K.; Cordan, J.; Güllülü, S.; Tuncel, E.; Baran, İ., et al. Effects of Origanum onites on Endothelial Function and Serum Biochemical Markers in Hyperlipidaemic Patients. Journal of International Medical Research 2008, 36, 1326-1334.

Coriander/Cilantro

Nichol, C. (2015). Essential spices and herbs: discover them, understand them, enjoy them. Berkeley, CA: Rockridge Press.

"Coriander." Our Herb Garden, 17 Mar. 2013, www.ourherbgarden.com/herb-history/coriander.html.

Hoxworth, Martin. "Coriandrum Sativum, Coriander." Camstar Herbs, www.camstar.co.uk/en/en/products/herbinfo/coriander.

Waheed, A.; Miana, G.; Ahmad, S.; Khan, M.A. Clinical investigation of hypoglycemic effect of Coriandrum sativum in type-2 (NIDDM) diabetic patients. Pakistan Journal of Pharmacology 2006, 23, 7-11.

Rajeshwari, C.; Andallu, B. Oxidative stress in NIDDM patients: influence of coriander (Coriandrum sativum) seeds. Res J Pharmaceut, Biol Chem Sci 2011, 2, 31-41.

Parsacyan, N. The effect of coriander seed powder consumption on atherosclerotic and cardioprotective indices of type 2 diabetic patients 2. Research 2012, 4, 86-90.

Rajeshwari, U.; Shobha, I.; Andallu, B. Comparison of aniseeds and coriander seeds for antidiabetic, hypolipidemic and antioxidant activities. Spatula DD-Peer Reviewed Journal on Complementary Medicine and Drug Discovery 2011, 1, 9-16.

Zahmatkesh, M.; Khodashenas-Roudsari, M. Comparing the therapeutic effects of three herbal medicine (cinnamon, fenugreek, and coriander) on hemoglobin A1C and blood lipids in type II diabetic patients. Chronic Diseases Journal 2013, 1, 74-82.

Rosemary

Sinkovic, A.; Suran, D.; Lokar, L.; Fliser, E.; Skerget, M.; Novak, Z.; Knez, Z. Rosemary extracts improve flow-mediated dilatation of the brachial artery and plasma PAI-1 activity in healthy young volunteers. Phytotherapy Research 2011, 25, 402-407.

Moore, J.; Yousef, M.; Tsiani, E. Anticancer Effects of Rosemary (Rosmarinus officinalis L.) Extract and Rosemary Extract Polyphenols. Nutrients 2016, 8, 731.

Cumin

Mercola. "What Are the Benefits and Uses of Cumin?" Mercola.com, articles.mercola.com/herbs-spices/cumin.aspx.

Wells, Katie. "Cumin for Digestion, Immune Health, & More | Wellness Mama." Wellness Mama®, 14 Oct. 2017, wellnessmama.com/5607/cumin-herb-profile/.

Taghizadeh, M.; Memarzadeh, M.R.; Asemi, Z.; Esmaillzadeh, A. Effect of the cumin cyminum Intake on Weight Loss, Metabolic Profiles and Biomarkers of Oxidative Stress in Overweight Subjects: A Randomized Double-Blind Placebo-Controlled Clinical Trial. Annals of Nutrition and Metabolism 2015, 66, 117-124.

Samani, K.G.; Farrokhi, E. Effects of cumin extract on oxLDL, paraoxanase 1 activity, FBS, total cholesterol, triglycerides, HDL-C, LDL-C, Apo A1, and Apo B in in the patients with hypercholesterolemia. International Journal of Health Sciences 2014, 8, 39-43.

Zare, R.; Heshmati, F.; Fallahzadeh, H.; Nadjarzadeh, A. Effect of cumin powder on body composition and lipid profile in overweight and obese women. Complementary Therapies in Clinical Practice 2014, 20, 297-301.

Andallu, B.; Ramya, V. Antihyperglycemic, cholesterol-lowering and HDL-raising effects of cumin (Cuminum cyminum) seeds in type-2 diabetes. Journal of Natural remedies 2007, 7, 142-149.
Jafari, S.; Mehdizadeh, A.; Ghavamzadeh, S. The Effect of Two Different Doses of Cuminum Cyminum Extract on Serum Glycemic Indices and Inflammatory Factors in Patients with Diabetes Type II: A Randomized Double-Blind Controlled Clinical Trial. Journal of Ardabil University of Medical Sciences 2016, 16, 200-210.

Jessica Elizabeth, D.L.T.; Gassara, F.; Kouassi, A.P.; Brar, S.K.; Belkacemi, K. Spice use in food: Properties and benefits. Critical Reviews in Food Science and Nutrition 2017, 57, 1078-1088.

Thyme

Dunn, Beth. "A Brief History of Thyme." History.com, A&E Television Networks, 10 May 2013, www.history.com/news/hungry-history/a-brief-history-of-thyme.

"Thyme." Our Herb Garden, 27 Jan. 2015, www.ourherbgarden.com/herb-history/thyme.html.

"The History of Thyme | Myspicer | Wholesale Spices & Herbs." MySpicer | Spices, Herbs, Seasonings, Rocky Mountain Spice Company, 28 May 2015, www.myspicer.com/the-history-of-thyme/.

"Thyme." The Epicentre, theepicentre.com/spice/thyme/.

Singletary, K. Thyme: History, Applications, and Overview of Potential Health Benefits. Nutrition Today 2016, 51, 40-49.

Mendez-Del Villar, M.; Puebla-Perez, A.M.; Sanchez-Pena, M.J.; Gonzalez-Ortiz, L.J.; Martinez-Abundis, E.; Gonzalez-Ortiz, M. Effect of Artemisia dracunculus Administration on Glycemic Control, Insulin Sensitivity, and Insulin Secretion in Patients with Impaired Glucose Tolerance. J Med Food 2016, 19, 481-485.

Cardamom

Nagdeve, Meenakshi. "11 Amazing Benefits of Cardamom." Organic Facts, 25 Oct. 2017, www.organicfacts.net/health-benefits/herbs-and-spices/health-benefits-of-cardamom.html.

Verma, S.K.; Jain, V., Singh, D.P. Effect of greater cardamom (Amomum subulatum Roxb.) on blood lipids, fibrinolysis and total antioxidant status in patients with ischemic heart disease. Asian Pacific Journal of Tropical Disease 2012, 2, S739-S743.

Fenugreek

"Brief History of the Fenugreek Herb." Brief History of the Fenugreek Herb, 28 July 2015, www.mdidea.com/products/herbextract/fenugreek. https://www.myspicer.com/history-of-fenugreek/.

Neelakantan, N.; Narayanan, M.; de Souza, R.J.; van Dam, R.M. Effect of fenugreek (Trigonella foenum-graecumL.) intake on glycemia: a meta-analysis of clinical trials. Nutrition Journal 2014, 13, 1-11.

Gupta, A.; Gupta, R.; Lal, B. Effect of Trigonella foenum-graecum (fenugreek) seeds on glycaemic control and insulin resistance in type 2 diabetes mellitus: a double blind placebo controlled study. J Assoc Physicians India 2001, 49.

Bordia, A.; Verma, S.K.; Srivastava, K.C. Effect of ginger (Zingiber officinale Rosc.) and fenugreek (Trigonella foenumgraecum L.) on blood lipids, blood sugar and platelet aggregation in patients with coronary artery disease. Prostaglandins Leukot Essent Fatty Acids 1997, 56.

Gong, J.; Fang, K.; Dong, H.; Wang, D.; Hu, M.; Lu, F. Effect of Fenugreek on Hyperglycaemia and Hyperlipidemia in Diabetes and Prediabetes: a Meta-analysis. Journal of Ethnopharmacology.

Sage

"Sage Benefits & Information (Salvia Officinalis)." Herbwisdom, www.herbwisdom.com/herb-sage.html.

Mateljan, George. Sage, www.whfoods.com/genpage.php?tname=foodspice&dbid=76.

"Smudge Stick." Wikipedia, Wikimedia Foundation, 28 Sept. 2017, en.wikipedia.org/wiki/Smudge_stick.

Kianbakht, S.; Abasi, B.; Perham, M.; Hashem Dabaghian, F. Antihyperlipidemic Effects of Salvia officinalis L. Leaf Extract in Patients with Hyperlipidemia: A Randomized Double-Blind Placebo-Controlled Clinical Trial. Phytotherapy Research 2011, 25, 1849-1853.

Sá, C.; Ramos, A.; Azevedo, M.; Lima, C.; Fernandes-Ferreira, M.; Pereira-Wilson, C. Sage Tea Drinking Improves Lipid Profile and Antioxidant Defences in Humans. International Journal of Molecular Sciences 2009, 10, 3937.

Behradmanesh, S.; Derees, F.; Rafieian-kopaei, M. Effect of Salvia officinalis on diabetic patients. Journal of Renal Injury Prevention 2013, 2, 51-54.

Kianbakht, S.; Dabaghian, F.H. Improved glycemic control and lipid profile in hyperlipidemic type 2 diabetic patients consuming Salvia officinalis L. leaf extract: A randomized placebo. Controlled clinical trial. Complementary therapies in medicine 2013, 21, 441-446.

Tarragon

"Tarragon." Our Herb Garden, Our Herb Garden 2008 - 2017, 17 Mar. 2013, www.ourherbgarden.com/herb-history/tarragon.html.

S.L., Botanical-online. "Tarragon Properties as a Spice." Botanical-Online, www.botanical-online.com/english/tarragon_spice.htm.

Mercola, Joseph. "Tarragon: Benefits, Uses and Recipes." Mercola.com, articles.mercola.com/herbs-spices/tarragon.aspx.

"Tarragon." A Modern Herbal | Tarragon, www.botanical.com/botanical/mgmh/t/tarrag07.html.

Bloomer, R.J.; Canale, R. Effect of an aqueous Russian tarragon extract on glucose tolerance in response to an oral dextrose load in non-diabetic men. Nutrition and Dietary Supplements 2011, 3, 43-49.

Nutmeg

"The History Of Nutmeg." InDepthInfo, www.indepthinfo.com/nutmeg/history.shtml.

"The History of Nutmeg | MySpicer.com | Spices, Herbs & Blends." MySpicer | Spices, Herbs, Seasonings, 4 Feb. 2014, www.myspicer.com/history-of-nutmeg/.

Saffron

Bathaie, S. Zahra. "Historical Uses of Saffron: Identifying Potential New Avenues for Modern Research." Academia.edu, www.academia.edu/3515595/Historical_Uses_of_Saffron_Identifying_Pot ential_New_Avenues_for_Modern_Research.

Basil

Publications, Inc. Ogden. "Basil: Herbal Lore and Legends." Mother Earth Living, www.motherearthliving.com/Natural-Health/basil-herbal-lore-and-legends.

Gernot Katzer. "Spice Pages: Basil (Ocimum basilicum/sanctum/tenuiflorum/canum)". gernot-katzers-spice-pages.com.

Father Kino's Herbs: Growing & Using them Today, 2011 Jacqueline A. Soule, Ph. D., Tierra del Sol Institute Press, Tucson, AZ.

"Basil." Wikipedia, Wikimedia Foundation, 29 Oct. 2017, en.wikipedia.org/wiki/Basil.

"Basil Ocimum Basilicum." Basil Herb Benefits, www.anniesremedy.com/ocimum-basilicum-basil.php?gc=4&gclid=CK3v0_XD89QCFQUNaQodRcMFeg.

Dill

Rashidlamir, A.; Gholamian, S.; Javaheri, A.H.; Dastani, M. The effect of 4-weeks aerobic training according with the usage of Anethum graveolens on blood sugar and lipoproteins profile of diabetic women. Annals of Biological Research 2012, 3, 4313-4319.

Mirhosseini, M.; Baradaran, A.; Rafeian-Kopaei, M. Anethum graveolens and hyperlipidemia: A randomized clinical trial. Journal of Research in Medical Sciences 2014, 19.

Mansouri, M.; Nayebi, N.; keshtkar, A.; Hasani-Ranjbar, S.; Taheri, E.; Larijani, B. The effect of 12 weeks Anethum graveolens (dill) on metabolic markers in patients with metabolic syndrome; a randomized double blind controlled trial. DARU Journal of Pharmaceutical Sciences 2012, 20, 1-7.

Sahib, A.S.; Mohammad, I.H.; Al-Gareeb, A.I. Effects of Anethum graveolens leave powder on lipid profile in hyperlipidemic patients. Spatula DD 2012, 2, 153-158.

Storing Spices

Madmone, Shuli. "Spice." WholeSpice, wholespice.com/blog/storing-and-keeping-your spices-fresh/.

Schettler, Renee. "The Best Way to Store Herbs." Real Simple, © 2017 Time Inc. Lifestyle Group, www.realsimple.com/food-recipes/shopping-storing/herbs-spices/best-way-store-herbs.

Revell, Janice. "Food Storage - How Long Can You Keep..." StillTasty: Your Ultimate Shelf Life Guide - Save Money, Eat Better, Help The Environment, www.stilltasty.com/Fooditems/index/17263.

Weight loss section references

Ramallal, R; Toledo, E; Martinez, JA: Shivappa, N; Hebert, J; Martinez-Gonzalez, MA; Ruiz-Canela, M. Inflammatory Potential of Diet, Weight Gain, and Incidence of Overweight/Obesity: The SUN Cohort. *Obesity*. 2017, 24, 997-1005.

Jungbauer, A; Medjakovic, S. Anti-inflammatory properties of culinary herbs and spices that ameliorate the effects of metabolic syndrome. *Maturitas*. 2012, 71, 227-239.

Mozaffari-Khosravi, H; Talaei, B; Jalali, BA; Najarzadeh, A; Mozayan, MR. The effect of ginger powder supplementation on insulin resistance and glycemic indices in patients with type 2 diabetes: a randomized, double-blind, placebo-controlled trial. *Complement Ther Med*. 2014, 22, 9-16.

Jagtap, S; Khare, P; Mangal, P; Kondepudi, KK; Bishnoi, M; Bhutani, KK. Effect of mahanimbine, an alkaloid from curry leaves, on high-fat diet-induced adiposity, insulin resistance, and inflammatory alterations. *Biofactors*. 2017, 43, 220-231.

Wang, S; Moustaid-Moussa, N; Chen, L; Mo, H; Shastri, A; Su, R; Bapat; P, Kwun, I; Shen, CL. Novel insights of dietary polyphenols and obesity. *J Nutr Biochem*. 2014, 25, 1-18.

Whitting, S; Derbyshire, E; Tiwari, BK. Capsaicinoids and capsinoids. A potential role for weight management? A systematic review of the evidence. *Appetite.* 2012, 59, 341-8.

Baothman, OA; Zamzami, MA; Taher, I; Abubaker, J; Abu-Farha, M. The role of gut microbiota in the development of obesity and Diabetes. *Lipids Health Dis.* 2016, 18, 108-15.

Mansour, MS; Ni, YM; Roberts, AL; Kelleman, M; Roychoudhury, A; St-Onge, MP. Ginger consumption enhances the thermic effect of food and promotes feelings of satiety without affecting metabolic and hormonal parameters in overweight men: a pilot study. *Metabolism.* 2012, 61, 1347-52.

Taghizadeh, M; Farzin, N; Taheri, S; Mahlouji, M; Akbari, H; Karamali, F; Asemi, Z. The effect of dietary supplements containing green tea, capsaicin, and ginger extracts on weight loss and metabolic profiles in overweight women: A randomized double-blind placebo-controlled clinical trial. *Ann Nutr Metab.* 2017, 70, 277-285.

Qing-Yi, L; Summanen, P; Ru-Po, L; Huang, J; Henning, S; Heber, D; Finegold, S; Li, Z. Prebiotic potential and chemical composition of seven culinary spice extracts. *Journal of Food Science.* 2017, 82, 1807-1813.

RECIPE INDEX

Basic Red Sauce, 60-61

Basic Spiced Morning
Muffin, 73

Basic Yogurt Dip, 61

Better Hemp Pesto, 97

Better Turmeric Pear Toast,
98

Black Bean Brownies, 129

Brazilian-Style Grilled
Chicken with *Chimichurri*, 124

Broccoli Cheese Frittata, 107

Cardamom Roast Pears with
Maple Yogurt, 78

Chef Neal's Famous Creole
Seasoning, 123

Cinnamon Almond Coffee,
126

Cinnamon Applesauce, 77

Cumin-Crusted Salmon Over
Silky Sweet Potatoes, 99

Curried Chicken with
Cucumber, 88

Curried Red Snapper with
Quinoa and Blanched Chard,
80

Deborah Parker Wong's
Spice and Wine Pairings, 128

Dr. Sanjay Gupta's Calming
Turmeric Tea, 90

Dr. Sears Vegetable Spice
Medley, 119

Exotic Spicy Tamarind-
Cauliflower Soup, 84

Ginger Fried Rice, 112

Gelman's More is More
Guacamole, 85

Greek Chicken Marinade, 109

Haydari – Turkish Yogurt Dip, 131

Heirloom Tomato and Smokey Chipotle Soup, 71

Herb Parmesan Crisp, 62

Herbed Salmon, 79

Hot and Spicy Fruit Salad, 71

Ikarian Cauliflower with Ginger & Fenugreek, 96

Kitchari, 86

Lemon-Barley Pilaf with Chicken and Thyme, 101

Lentil Soup, 130

Lentil with Herb Roasted Vegetable Soup, 68

Lentils Three Ways: Soup, Side, & Salad, 89

Macerated Strawberries, 91

Maque Choux, 122

Mediterranean Chow-Chow, 121

Moroccan Turkey Chili, 110

Mushroom with Fresh Thyme Soup, 69

Mustard Spiced Salmon Filets, 65

My Mom's Spicy Turkey

Chili, 67

Nectarine Relish, 62

Oven-Baked Swedish Meatballs, 113

Oven-Roasted Cod with Tomato Jam, Feta and Olives, 103

Pear Spice Smoothie, 115

Peruvian Chicken, 93

Quick Spiced Tomato Soup, 128

Quick Spiced Winter Soups, 128

Ricotta Pumpkin Cheesecake, 72

Saffron Herb Pistachio Rice, 95

Salmon Spice or Herb Kebabs, 65

Slow-Cooker Chicken Burrito Bonanza, 105

Spice Rubbed Grilled Chicken Dinner, 64

Spiced Pork Roast with Cauliflower Mash, 111

Spiced Quinoa, 66

Spiced Sweet Potato Bisque, 67

Spiced Walnuts, 92

Spicy Fish Tacos, 63

Spicy Grilled Pineapple, 116

Spicy Tofu with Black-Eyed
Peas and Braised Chard
Soup, 70

Stewed Blueberries, 86

Super Simple Spicy Soup,
127

Sweet Baked Apples with
Cherries and Citrus, 100

"Tagine" Style Chicken, Beef
or Eggplant, 117

Tomato Basil Dijon
Vinaigrette, 59

Tomato Curry Soup, 126

Turkey Burger with Ranch
Dressing, 107

Turmeric Chicken Soup, 76

Turmeric Latte, 126

Vivica's Tasty Tacos, 82

White Peach Ginger
Smoothie, 114

Working Moms 10 Minute
Chicken, 134

ABOUT THE AUTHORS

Melina B. Jampolis, MD is an internist and board certified physician nutrition specialist (one of only a several hundred practicing in the United States) and is the immediate past president of the National Board of Physician Nutrition Specialists. Trained as an internist, for the past 15 years she has specialized exclusively in nutrition for weight loss, disease prevention and treatment.

A graduate of Tufts University and Tufts School of Medicine, she completed her residency in Internal Medicine at Santa Clara Valley Medical Center, a Stanford University teaching hospital and became board certified as a physician nutrition specialist in 2004. In 2005, Dr. Melina hosted a program on the **Discovery Network's FIT TV** titled "Fit TV's Diet Doctor" and served as the diet and fitness expert **CNNHealth.com** from 2008-2014 and remains a consultant. She is the immediate past president of the National Board of Physician Nutrition Specialists and remains on the board of directors.

Her first book, *The No-Time-to-Lose-Diet*, was published in January 2007 by Nelson Books and the paperback version, *The Busy Person's Guide to Permanent Weight Loss* was released in May 2008. Her latest book, *The Calendar Diet – A month by month guide to losing weight while living your life*, was released in March 2012 by Wagging Tail Press and her third book, *The Doctor on Demand Diet* (Ghost Mountain Books, 2015) was released in November 2015. This book, *Spice Up, Slim Down* has been released in December 2017 by Wagging Tail Press and 100% of the profits will go to charity to fight childhood malnutrition around the world.

Her latest business venture, **SpiceFit**, is dedicated to producing the highest quality, research supported, spice based supplements for weight loss and achieving optimal health. A percentage of proceeds from this company will also go to charity as philanthropy has always been a core component of Dr. Melina's work. She is a member of the American Society of Nutrition, the Obesity Society, and the International Society and Nutrigenetics and Nutrigenomics.

Dr. Melina is frequent guest on popular TV shows including Live with Kelly, The Doctors, Dr. Oz. show, CNN, Hallmark Home & Family, and Fox News and Business Network and she has appeared on the Today show, Access Hollywood Live, The Talk, and numerous local television and radio stations including ABC, NBC, FOX, KGO radio and KRON-4 news.

She is highly sought after public speaker and consultant and she lectures and presents throughout the country on the topic of 'food as medicine' and nutrition for weight loss and optimal health. She serves on the scientific advisory board of several nutrition-focused companies and has recently joined UCLA Center for Human Nutrition to pursue research in the nutrition field.

She has done hundreds of print interviews including USA Today, USA Weekend, Us World & News Report, New York Post, Family Circle, Prevention, WashingtonPost.com, Better Homes & Gardens, Glamour.com, Forbes.com, Ladies Home Journal, First for Women, Women's World, Alternative Medicine Magazine, Women's Health,

Health, Clean Eating, Baby Talk, and more on nutrition and weight loss related topics.

Dr. Melina lives in Los Angeles with her husband and young sons and maintains a small private practice Los Angeles. She believes whole-heartedly in the role of nutrition in preventative medicine and achieving optimal health. She teaches a balanced and sustainable lifestyle based eating and exercise program and has helped thousands clients over the past two decades improve their health and well-being.

She is dedicated to the treatment and prevention of childhood obesity, particularly in the low income, minority population. Her volunteer work includes helping to launch a health food pantry in the Hunter's point neighborhood of San Francisco, and bi-weekly family nutrition and obesity counseling sessions at the Bresee Foundation in Los Angeles, a center for low income, minority children.

Dr. Kristina Petersen is an Accredited Practicing Dietitian and has a PhD in Nutritional Science from the University of South Australia. She is currently a Research Associate at The Pennsylvania State University and her research focuses on dietary components and patterns to improve risk factors for cardiometabolic disease. She is currently working on a clinical trial investigating the health benefits of herbs and spices, and previously she has conducted research exploring the cardiometabolic effects of fruits and vegetables, potassium rich foods, sodium, and the Mediterranean diet. She has published close to 30 peer reviewed articles on these topics and has presented the findings of her work at national and international conferences.